THE
PAIN
SURVIVAL
GUIDE

THE
PAIN SURVIVAL GUIDE

How to Reclaim Your Life

Dennis C. Turk, PhD
Frits Winter, PhD

American Psychological Association • Washington, DC

First printing, August 2005
Second printing, January 2008

Published by
APA LifeTools
750 First Street, NE
Washington, DC 20002
www.apa.org

To order
APA Order Department
P.O. Box 92984
Washington, DC 20090-2984
Tel: (800) 374-2721; Direct: (202) 336-5510
Fax: (202) 336-5502; TDD/TTY: (202) 336-6123
Online: www.apa.org/books/
E-mail: order@apa.org

In the U.K., Europe, Africa, and the Middle East, copies may be ordered from
American Psychological Association
3 Henrietta Street
Covent Garden, London
WC2E 8LU England

Typeset in Garamond by World Composition Services, Inc., Sterling, VA

Printer: Port City Press, Inc., Baltimore, MD
Cover Designer: Naylor Design, Washington, DC
Technical/Production Editor: Dan Brachtesende

The opinions and statements published are the responsibility of the authors, and such opinions and statements do not necessarily represent the policies of the American Psychological Association.

Library of Congress Cataloging-in-Publication Data
Turk, Dennis C.
 The pain survival guide : how to reclaim your life / Dennis C. Turk and Frits Winter.—1st ed.
  p. cm.
 ISBN 1-59147-049-8
 1. Chronic pain. 2. Pain—Psychological aspects. I. Winter, Frits. II. Title.
 RB127.T872 2005
 616'.0472—dc22   2005006585

British Library Cataloguing-in-Publication Data
A CIP record is available from the British Library.

Printed in the United States of America

To all of our patients who have taught us so much about what it means to be a person with pain and not just a pain patient.

Contents

THE
PAIN
SURVIVAL
GUIDE

Introduction: How This Program Can Change Your Life

*I*f you feel pain much of the time or if you have repeated episodes of severe pain, you are aware of how it affects the quality of your entire life. Perhaps only you know the favorite activities you have given up, the outings you've declined, even the friends you have lost because of your pain-induced limitations.

Perhaps you have tried medical treatments such as prescription drugs, physical therapy, or even surgery. When these have led to limited success, your health care providers may have told you, "*We've done all we can, you will just have to learn to live with it.*" This dismissive comment is very disheartening because you do not want to live with your pain. You had been living with your pain for too long even before you sought treatment. Rather, you want to live *without* it!

If these practitioners had told you *how* you can live with pain in a way that allows you to reclaim your life, that might have been a different story. If they had told you how you could bring quality and happiness back into your life by taking simple steps consistently, you might have had realistic hope again.

That is where this program begins—with the restoration of hope. By following a program that is deceptively simple, free, and clinically proven, you will, day by day and week by week, reclaim your life. Each of the self-management lessons in this book is backed by research and has been clinically proven to help people with chronic health conditions, especially chronic pain, to reduce their symptoms and restore the quality of their lives.

In this book, we will help you change your feelings of hopelessness and helplessness into realistic hope and empowerment. If your doctors have thrown up their hands and said that your case is "hopeless" or "treatment resistant," we hope to help you prove them wrong. Most important, we will help you begin to really live again!

Why Not Seek More Medical Treatment Now?

When you stand in line at supermarkets and see the headlines of tabloid papers announcing new cures for arthritis, cancer, and other pain-inducing diseases, it is hard to turn away. But when you then consider these claims in the context of the tabloid also announcing new sightings of Elvis, alien abductions, and ways to lose 25 pounds in 5 days (with no effort, of course), you may reconsider.

However, when you see mainstream newspapers describing transplants of all kinds of complex organs and new heart disease surgeries, you may more reasonably think, "Surely there must be a new treatment for my pain. Perhaps I should see the doctor again." This is understandable. We all want to believe that when we have a problem in our lives, there is someone out there who can fix it. No one suggests that there is no hope for your car when, after you have taken it in to the mechanic, it has problems again. People tell you to take the car back to the mechanic or get a new mechanic. They never suggest that the problem is "all in your head" or is somehow your fault, as some people do when they hear you suffer from chronic pain.

So why shouldn't you look to a different doctor, or perhaps undertake a different surgery, or try a new drug? It is always good to get a second opinion when you have chronic pain. However, if you have seen more than two doctors who are up-to-date on recent medical advances in pain, going to a third or fourth doctor is likely to cause more frustration and feelings of hopelessness.

We are not suggesting that there may *never* be a way to reduce your pain by newly discovered drugs or surgical treatment. Over the last decade, there have been many advances in medicine for some pain conditions. However, despite these developments, there is currently no treatment that can eliminate *all pain* for *all people all of the time*. Even the most powerful treatments (namely, opioid drugs, anticonvulsant and antidepressant medications, and surgery) typically reduce pain by no more than 40%. Only rarely is pain eliminated by currently available treatments. There may be breakthroughs tomorrow, but right now it makes more sense to become your own pain expert and begin to manage your pain and your life.

When Friends and Family Don't Help

When you have chronic pain, you may get the feeling that not only your doctor but even your closest family and friends do not realize what it feels like to have chronic pain 24 hours a day, 365 days a year or to experience frequent devastating acute pain at unpredictable times. Unlike when you have the flu and people can see your symptoms, pain is maddeningly invisible to anyone else but the sufferer. There is simply no pain thermometer that you can show to someone to prove that you are ill.

Some family members or friends may subtly (or not so subtly) insinuate that you are exaggerating the extent and depth of your pain or your pain-induced limitations. The truly uninformed may suspect that you just want to gain attention, elicit sympathy, avoid responsibilities, or receive disability payments. Such responses can elicit feelings of undeserved shame. And, they definitely add to feelings of frustration, anger, and depression. It is helpful to know that everyone feels bad when his or her concerns are not taken seriously.

So What Should You Do Now?

Do you remember the Peanuts cartoon strip in which Charlie Brown is standing on the baseball mound talking to Lucy? He wonders if he should play baseball that day as his arm hurts, his stomach hurts, and his back hurts. Lucy advises, "**Play anyway! Don't let your body push you around!**"

As you will see later in this book, it is not always wise to "play anyway" (although it is always wise to play!). But Lucy's other point is totally in line with our thinking. We will not provide a miracle "cure," but we will help you learn how "not to let your body push you around." We will be your coaches, and we will help you enlist people in your life to be on your team. This will ensure that you, not your pain, are in charge of your life.

Perhaps even those people whose remarks elicited feelings of shame or anger in the past will be on your team once they see that you take your pain seriously enough to make managing it your first priority. Perhaps when they see the efforts you are making, they will finally realize that your pain is real, after all. And, even if they don't, *you* will feel better. *You* will take up some of your favorite activities again. And *you* will feel realistic hope, perhaps for the first time in years.

Are we exaggerating? You will be the ultimate judge of that. But we promise that we are offering you a clinically proven program that has been used successfully with thousands of people just like you. A great deal of research evidence exists to support our confidence in our approach to a wide variety of pain problems—back pain, fibromyalgia, chronic headache, arthritis, and many more. (At the end of the book we have included a representative list of published studies on which we based our program, should you be interested in the scientific findings behind each of our lessons.)

There are two things we must tell you, however. First, our program comes with a warning label. As with instructions on labels of antibiotic drugs, you must "take all the treatment in the book (bottle)" to reap the full benefits.

Second, this program is relatively simple. But, simple does not necessarily mean easy. We know of no "easy" way to manage chronic pain. It just does not exist. You will need to make pain management an important priority in your life. Worked consistently, these lessons can help you thrive.

An Overview of Our Program

This program consists of ten related lessons. Each has a specific focus, but all are designed to help you gain control of your pain and your life. In fact, if these lessons are put into practice consistently, they can help you thrive!

In lesson 1, you will learn about pain in general, about the enormous number of people who suffer from pain, and about the incapacitating effects of chronic pain. You will learn that you are not alone. For example, surveys have shown that up to one third of the population of the United States has some form of chronic or recurring pain problem. Most important, you will also learn some of the erroneous and harmful **myths** about pain. Believing these myths as if they were facts will interfere with your ability to gain control over your pain. Knowledge is the true beginning of power.

In lesson 2, you will learn to recognize the first important pain reducer: **optimal activity, rest,** and **pacing.** Rather than remaining immobile or pushing yourself too hard, you will learn how to find a proper balance between exertion and rest. You will learn the importance of pacing your activities to prevent increased pain while still being able to enjoy being active. Practicing will enable you to gradually increase your energy, activities, and conditioning without harming yourself or making your pain worse.

In lesson 3, you will learn to recognize the value of the second key pain reducer—**relaxation**. This relaxation is not the kind in which you put your feet up and watch television in a haze. You're probably bored with that by now anyway, even if you may want to deny this at times. Instead, you will learn how you can create deep relaxation, beneficial rest, and hence enjoy many activities that you may not have considered before.

In lesson 4, we discuss the problems of chronic tiredness and disturbed sleep that many of our patients experience. We share with you our best knowledge of how to defeat chronic fatigue and achieve a good night's rest. As you *consistently* practice lessons 2, 3, and 4, you will notice a reduction in your experience of pain, and passively watching television will be even *more* boring!

Up to this point, you've been working alone with us, your coaches. In lesson 5, you will learn how you can include other people in your life as teammates. We teach you to communicate with others in your life in such a way that they will support and encourage you. If they are stubborn, we help you to find new people who can provide understanding and support and help you make the most of this program. You may not need a whole baseball team, but you do need at least one or two people to cheer you on. Even if you consider yourself a loner, you should know that understanding, acceptance, and support are proved pain reducers.

In lesson 6, we focus on changing behavior (your own especially) by learning about the laws of learning. We will teach you a number of principles with which you can influence your own behavior and (sometimes) that of others (and vice versa). You will learn how the behaviors and responses of others affect you, even without your being aware of this. You will also learn how to change certain aspects of your lifestyle that contribute to (note that we do not say *cause*) or worsen your pain.

In lesson 7, we focus on how you think and feel when you experience pain. We know you are not creating your pain by your thoughts and emotional reactions. But you can help control your pain by changing how you think about and react to it. You will learn how you can influence and control your mental and emotional responses to the very real pain you are experiencing. You will be able to direct your thoughts and feelings so that they contribute to your sense of control rather than to feelings of helplessness and hopelessness.

In lesson 8, you will learn to regain self-confidence and to trust yourself again. With regard to trust, this may seem odd. We usually think of trust as having to do with other people. However, people with chronic pain often lose trust in their bodies and hence themselves. If others are not supportive (and we include some health care practitioners here), you may lose trust in others as well. Trust, especially in yourself, and self-confidence are potent factors in managing pain. You will learn coping skills and problem-solving strategies to regain self-trust and self-confidence. These will allow you to further control your pain.

In lesson 9, you will learn more about the relation between your pain and how your daily habits may be influence your perception of pain. You will also learn how your past experiences affect your relationship with pain now. You will learn to identify and change more things in your life that are contributing to the negative effects of your pain.

If you have reached lesson 10 and worked each lesson diligently, you will be much happier and will have taken on many activities you never thought you would do again. However, it is just as important to learn to maintain these gains. In lesson 10, we help you continue your self-management program, manage setbacks and relapses, and maintain the benefits you have achieved. As you learn that you can bounce back, you will be even more likely to confront and seek out new challenges. You will learn how to stay motivated for life!

We strongly encourage you to keep some kind of diary or journal as you work through the lessons in this program. At the end of each lesson, we have included a set of questions for you to consider or exercises for you to complete. We have designed each "homework assignment" exercise to help you learn specific skills and ways to control your pain. You don't have to do all of them. We will indicate which questions and activities are critical by putting them in **boldface** type. However, we encourage you to at least try one or two others as well. Perhaps you can pick the one that appeals most to you. Some of our patients, however, have gained the most from choosing the one question or exercise that they least wanted to answer or do. Participating in this way will help you relate the information in the lesson to your own unique circumstances.

Most important are our suggestions for keeping track of your progress. The charts we introduce in lessons 2 and 3 should be photocopied and kept in your journal or in a notebook on an ongoing basis. These records are critical because improvements can be so gradual that you may not know you are improving unless you have a record to look back on. Also, you may have heard that keeping a food diary has been shown to be *a* if not *the* critical component in most weight-reduction programs. The same is true for reducing pain; keeping track of your efforts can help you get on track and stay on track over the long haul.

At the end of the book we also include a list of suggested additional reading, organized by lesson. These readings are optional, but they may help you when your motivation is lagging. Most of the books listed can be obtained from libraries or bookstores in your community or through the Internet.

A Note of Encouragement Before Beginning

One of the many people who has consistently followed our program was asked what her biggest achievement was. She said,

> Before the program, I got up with the thought, "Heavens, another long, painful day. I wish it were evening again."
> In the evening in bed I thought, "Heavens, another long, painful night, I wish it were morning again. In my darkest hours I even thought that perhaps it would be better if I did not see the morning again."
> I knew that this was not living. I didn't want to grow old like this.
> After consistently following this program, I now sleep reasonably well, enjoy friends, family, and activities, and when I wake up, I look forward to the new day.

Another of our patients said,

> The desire to continue living and being able to feel a considerable degree of control over pain is the greatest achievement of my life, outside of raising my children.

Men, who often say similar things in fewer words, also have encouragement to share. As one patient said,

> I'm a new man now; I've regained my life.

If you are ready to live again, let's get started.

Becoming Your Own Pain Management Expert

"Grant me the serenity to accept the things I cannot change,
courage to change the things I can,
and wisdom to know the difference."
—Serenity Prayer, Rheinhold Neibuhr

*E*veryone has pain at times. The reassuring thing about most pain is that it will usually go away with time. A sports injury and its resulting pain, such as an elbow injured during a casual game of tennis, will eventually heal with resting that part of the arm. Once the pain has ceased for the weekend tennis player, the suffering is soon forgotten.

For most people, it is unthinkable that pain will never go away. That is part of why they don't understand the plight of those who experience chronic pain.

Even those with chronic pain don't like to think of it as such. If we admit to having chronic pain, it means admitting it will last a long time or perhaps will never go away at all. It's scary to think that way, and such thinking can also make the pain seem even worse.

If doctors have been stymied and called your pain "treatment-resistant" or "chronic," you may have asked yourself, "Have the doctors been defeated by my pain? "Have they given up on me?" Am I condemned to a life of inactivity, anger, helplessness, suffering, and despair?" These are normal but very depressing thoughts!

The good news is that many thousands of people have proved that despite the presence of pain, they do not have to give in and give up control of their lives. They have found a middle ground. They are not denying that their pain is chronic, but they are also stepping up to the plate and confronting their pain. They have found a balance between acceptance and change. The Serenity Prayer with which we began this lesson seems particularly applicable, especially the words *serenity, courage,* and most important, *wisdom.*

Our patients begin to no longer think of themselves as patients but rather as pain self-managers. They have gradually learned what they are capable of doing, and they have done that and gained even more capability. Although once pain held them completely in its grip, they have found ways to overcome its debilitating effects. They have become smarter, more clever, and wiser. They have gained control over their pain and their lives. As you work through this book, it will become clear to you that while others can support you, you must become your own expert on your pain and your own pain manager.

In the coming lessons, we will coach you to become that expert. You already know more than you think. Nobody knows your pain as well as you do, not even the finest doctors in the world. Nor does your neighbor with a similar ailment know your pain as well as you know it, because pain is an incredibly *personal* experience.

It is your personal expertise in pain that will be our basis in coaching you. It will help us to help you design a plan to manage your pain, which is as unique as you are. In this lesson, you will learn more about pain so that you can better understand your own. Knowledge is power!

The Nature of Chronic Pain

We have used the phrase *chronic pain* several times already in this book, but what exactly defines pain as chronic? Usually, pain following overuse or injury is considered to be chronic when it continues to interfere with living or does not become much less intense after the expected period of healing (i.e., medical estimates as to how long it takes for tissue damage to heal following an injury or overuse). Pain is also considered chronic when it is related to a progressive disease (such as arthritis or cancer).

For most acute injuries, such as as a sprained ankle, the expected period of healing is from several weeks to several months. For back injuries, the pain may last longer, but with proper care should remit over a period of time. For pain following minor surgery, the expected period of healing might only be a few days.

Thus, there is no exact time at which pain ceases to be acute and becomes chronic. But most of us know when we have a chronic disease such as arthritis. We also tend to know when pain from an injury has persisted well beyond the expected course. And, we can all agree that pain has become chronic when it alters our lifestyle and serves no useful purpose (more about the purpose of pain later in this lesson).

Chronic Pain Is Very Common—All Too Common!

When we have chronic pain, it is easy to feel as if we are alone. The reality is, however, that chronic pain is unfortunately very common. Recent surveys provide some rather surprising, and to many distressing, information (see Exhibit 1.1).

Exhibit 1.1. The Magnitude of the Problem

In the United States alone,

- ◆ over 11 million people experience migraine headaches;
- ◆ 23 million people report the presence of chronic back pain;
- ◆ 37 million people indicate they have pain associated with arthritis;
- ◆ 3 to 6 million people are diagnosed with fibromyalgia;
- ◆ 3.5 million people experience pain associated with cancer and its treatment;
- ◆ annual costs (health care, disability, lost productivity) of chronic pain may exceed $125 billion this year.

Although pain is a personal experience, you have a lot of company when it comes to experiencing chronic pain. Of course, knowing that such large numbers of others experience chronic pain does not diminish your suffering. But at least there is some solace in knowing that you are not alone. And there is even more solace in knowing that many of these people have learned to live fulfilling lives despite their pain. You can too!

The Usefulness of Pain

Acute pain can be useful as a warning that you have gone beyond your body's limitations, but the pain signaling system is unreliable at times. Often, harm is occurring within the body and no pain is experienced. Even more often, harm cannot be detected with classic medical tests, but pain is clearly present.

Harm, but No Pain

Often, people with cancer feel quite healthy until their disease progresses into a very serious condition. A lump that is not noticeable to anyone but a well-trained physician can be discovered during a routine medical check up and turn out to be malignant. The patient in question may feel no pain at all, and yet something life-threatening is occurring in his or her body. Following successful surgery or chemotherapy, he or she may still experience pain or other kinds of discomfort, but the pain is not caused by the tumor but by the treatment itself.

Likewise, there are a substantial number of people who do not report pain, but when diagnostic tests like x-rays are performed, significant pathology is present. In fact, studies have shown that when sophisticated diagnostic procedures (such as magnetic resonance images [MRIs], and computed axial tomography [CAT scans]), are performed, as many as 35% of people who have **no** reported symptoms and **no** pain at all, show significant physical pathology. This is pathology that we *might* reasonably expect to cause pain! Contrary to what we might believe, there is not a close relationship between the amount of pain we feel and the amount of harm occurring in our bodies. That's why it is important to have routine medical check ups!

Pain, but No Objective Evidence

There are many common chronic pain conditions such as back pain, whiplash (resulting from neck injuries frequently following motor vehicle accidents), fibromyalgia (a painful musculoskeletal condition characterized by widespread and persistent pain and fatigue), and migraine and tension headaches in which little evidence of physical pathology can be detected. For example, in up to 85% of people with back pain, doctors are unable to determine a physical cause. Yet, such pain may be severe, causing significant distress and disability. In the case of chronic headaches, there is rarely any identifiable tissue damage that can explain the experience of pain, yet these people suffer enormously. In whiplash injuries and fibromyalgia, no physical cause can be identified in a substantial majority of the people who report that their pain is severe and greatly diminishes the quality of their lives.

Some people for whom medical tests do not show a cause for their pain may be told outright that their pain is not real. Or, more often, they receive subtle signals from doctors, family members, or insurance claims managers that they are exaggerating normal aches and pains. You may have experienced such skepticism yourself. We do not agree with such messages. All pain is real to the person who experiences it!

Same Injury, Same Treatment, Different Results

Another puzzling aspect of pain is the fact that people with the same medical diagnosis (either injury or disease) often respond quite differently to identical treatments. For example, three people may have surgery for a problem that is apparently caused by a dysfunction of a spinal disc (such discs function as "shock absorbers" in the body). Following surgery, one patient is very happy because the pain is gone. Another is disappointed and surprised to find the pain feels the same. A third person is very distressed because the pain feels even worse than before the surgery. These are common experiences for people who have undergone disc surgery. The results suggest that factors other than damage to the disc, bones, nerves, and muscles associated with the spine must be contributing to the pain experienced after surgery.

Misleading Pain

There are also a number of pain disorders in which the pain system gives a misleading signal. You feel pain in one place, but the damage is someplace else. Doctors call this "referred" pain. The pain at one place in the body *refers* to damage somewhere else in the body. For example, pain on the side of the biceps in the arm may indicate a frozen shoulder syndrome. Back pain may be caused by problems in the stomach or pelvis.

Finally, there are "strange" pain experiences that occur following amputation or after damage to the spinal cord. Quite commonly, pain is felt *as if* it were in the amputated limb— a limb that is no longer attached to a body! This is referred to as *phantom-limb* pain. However, whereas the limb may be phantom, the pain certainly is not!

Pain is also frequently felt in the lower limbs of people who have had a spinal cord injury and are paralyzed. Some of these individuals experience real pain in their legs although they cannot move them. This pain is counterintuitive, because through damage to the spinal cord, the nerve pathways linking the spinal cord to the brain are completely severed. Theoretically, no messages signaling injury can travel along the nerves to ever reach the brain. Thus, there should be no pain signals registering in the brain and therefore, there should be no pain. Yet, a significant proportion of people with spinal cord injuries do, in fact, feel severe pain. How can this be? It is as if the plug has been pulled from the radio but the music is still playing. Pain is indeed one of the most mysterious of physical maladies.

Take Your Pain Seriously

Extreme pain is real, even if there is no "objective" (i.e., observable) cause for it as defined by current medical diagnostic techniques. The same is true for depression, for example. A person can be depressed or suicidal when his or her whole life is going well, and nothing will show up on any medical test. And this has been true for decades. The Russian author Tolstoy once wrote, "I am very rich and famous; millions of Russians read my books. I possess a big farm, a wife and five children and the only thought that haunts me is: shall I use a rope or a gun to end it all?"

Many people with chronic pain become depressed. They have to take that seriously as well as their pain and consult a mental health professional when these feelings interfere with their quality of life.

The same is true with anxiety. A person in no objective danger can break out in a sweat and feel as if he or she is going to die. That is why it is good to once again repeat that feelings of fear, sadness, and pain can be extremely intense, even if they seem out of proportion to the so-called *objective* facts. When chastising themselves for having pain and thinking of themselves as weak, individuals with anxiety or depression often think they are "going crazy."

Neither the pain sufferer nor the person suffering from anxiety or depression is weak or crazy. What they have in common is that they must search for a solution rather than focusing on what may or may not be the cause.

Seek the Solution, Not the Cause

In cases of chronic pain, both the sufferer and the doctor initially seek to find the cause of the pain. By this, doctors usually mean the physical cause. Long after a second opinion has been sought and the doctor has "given up," the patient may continue to try to find the cause of the pain.

However, the main question is not, *How or why did I get the pain?* The critical question is, *What can I do to manage my pain so that I can get on with my life?*

We will discuss the role of factors other than physical damage in pain later in this book. Here, we discuss some of them briefly in the context of Gate Control Theory.

The Gate Control Theory

Imagine a door or gate in your spinal cord. Before your pain became chronic or before you had a progressive disease such as arthritis, usually this gate was closed and you did not feel pain. If you had an injury or some other type of obvious physical damage occurred, signals were sent along your nerves (the wiring of our bodies) to the spinal cord. These signals opened the gate and allowed information about the injury or damage to your body to reach the brain. This is where these signals are interpreted, with the result being the feeling of pain. In these cases, as you healed sometimes the pain was better and sometimes it was worse. It depended on how far open or closed the gate was.

In Exhibit 1.2 we have included a summary of the different factors that are known to open and close the pain gate.

The idea of a pain gate that can be opened and closed will help you understand that pain, especially chronic pain, cannot simply be eliminated by cutting out a painful body part or cutting nerves. In the past, nerves were cut in the hope of blocking pain. Unfortunately, all too often the surgical procedures created more problems than they solved. The nervous system does not operate like a simple cable system that can just be clipped and repaired. It is a living system that is continually changing and adapting to new circumstances and new information.

In addition to this information, it's helpful to know about common folklore about pain that can actually decrease your chances of living a zestful life. A couple of these ideas we

Exhibit 1.2. Summary of the Factors That Can Open and Close the Pain Gate

Factors that can open the pain gate

◇ Physical factors

⇑ Extent of injury
⇑ Inappropriate activity level

◇ Emotional stress

⇑ Depression
⇑ Worry/fear
⇑ Tension
⇑ Anger

◇ Thoughts

⇑ Focusing on the pain
⇑ Boredom due to minimal involvement in life activities
⇑ Nonadaptive attitudes and expectations ("It will never end!" "I'm helpless and hopeless!")

Factors that can close the pain gate

◇ Physical factors

⇓ Medication
⇓ Counterstimulation (heat, rubbing)
⇓ Appropriate activity level
⇓ Rest

◇ Relative emotional stability

⇓ Relaxation
⇓ Positive emotions (happiness, optimism)

◇ Thoughts

⇓ Life involvement, increased interest in life activities
⇓ Concentration/distraction
⇓ Adaptive attitudes/positive thoughts and feelings ("I can control my feelings." "I can reduce my level of muscle tension." "I am capable of doing many things despite my pain.")

have already briefly discussed, but the information is so important to your recovery that it bears repeating.

Common Myths About Pain

Myth 1: Pain is ALWAYS a reliable signal of physical damage and injury. Pain may be a clear and reliable signal of damage to the body. When this occurs, pain is useful; it has a purpose, namely, protection. Pain makes it clear to you when the water in a bath is too hot; this information can prevent you from burning yourself. Such pain makes you feel uncomfortable when you are trying on shoes and they are too tight. The pain tells you not to buy them!

However, as discussed earlier, pain is not always a reliable indicator of where and to what extent harm is occurring in the body. Most important, pain, in the form of discomfort on exertion, is not necessarily an indicator for action or inaction when it comes to chronic pain. We will talk more about this important topic in the next lesson.

Myth 2: When no clear physical damage is found by diagnostic procedures, pain must be imaginary. If this were true, millions of people with back pain, headache, phantom-limb pain, and pain following spinal cord injuries would all be suffering from imaginary pain! An epidemic of imaginary pain is not very likely.

For too long, only when a direct relationship could be found between pain and visible damage was pain taken seriously. The absence of identifiable physical pathology does not negate pain and suffering, nor does it guarantee that no physical factors may be contributing to the pain. As noted earlier, all pain is real, regardless of what anyone else has told you.

Myth 3: Chronic pain that does not respond to standard treatment should not be taken seriously. Lack of knowledge and ignorance about chronic pain have caused great physical and emotional distress (anxiety, depression, frustration, anger) for many people. Too many individuals still believe that "You can only have pain and feel pain when your pain has been legitimized by a physician." This implies that only a doctor can determine whether you have a right to your feelings of pain. No one has a right to tell you what you are feeling, no matter how many academic degrees he or she may have.

Unfortunately, pain is not directly observable. It is an intensely personal experience. There is, as yet, no *pain thermometer* that measures the internal experience of pain. Only *you* know how much pain you feel and how often you feel it.

Myth 4: There is a pill for every ill. When in doubt, cut it out. People, particularly those in the United States, have been flooded with advertisements suggesting that there should be a "pill" for every problem. The print and television media reinforce this: *Can't sleep at night? Take a pill. Don't have enough energy? Take a pill. Feel upset? Take a pill. Prevent indigestion before eating a spicy meal. Take a pill.*

Now, surgery too is being recommended like never before. *If you don't like the way your face or body looks, have surgery. Think you look too fat? Have liposuction. Don't like your lips? Have collagen injections. Breasts too small or too large? Implants and breast reduction surgery to the rescue!* Even people with well-earned wrinkles are advised to have Botox treatments.

Depending on pills and surgery sounds so much better than learning what it takes to change your behavior or your mindset. We are not saying that medication and surgery are never appropriate. There is a time and place for medication and surgery. But the mass media are not qualified to make these decisions. Don't be brainwashed by their messages.

When it comes to pain, be informed. For example, every month there seems to be a new arthritis pill advertised on television. Some of these are just a variation on a medication for which the patent has just expired. What these advertisements don't tell you is that even the most potent pain medications produce only about a 35% reduction of pain and in only about one-half of the people who take them! And taking medication definitely does not ensure long-term improvements in quality of life.

Myth 5: Pain is a signal to stop moving. In instances of pain following an acute injury or trauma (e.g., a broken leg as a result of a fall from a ladder), it may be appropriate to desist from activities that increase pain. In these cases, the pain is serving as a reliable warning signal. Remember the joke about the man who goes to a doctor and says, "Doc, it hurts when I do this." The doctor replies "Don't do that!"

However, for people with chronic pain, feeling pain or discomfort with exertion is not a reliable signal to cease activity. In fact, some forms of inactivity increase pain in chronic pain patients (more about this later). Consider that even following heart surgery, doctors recommend certain activities because being active tends to speed recovery—although it hurts at first!

For those with chronic pain, discomfort following reasonable activities may have little to do with the original cause of the pain and more to do with reduction in strength, endurance, and flexibility of muscles due to lack of use. In the next lesson, we will describe guidelines for how to increase activity to eventually decrease pain. But for now keep in mind that *not moving* may be increasing your pain and disability over time.

Myth 6: If you have had pain for a long time and doctors have told you that they have "done all they can," your situation is hopeless. This is perhaps the most dangerous myth we have described. It undermines your efforts to gain control over your pain and your life. As this book will show, everyone can make changes that lead to pain reduction and improved quality of life.

Treatments for Pain

Many of you know the most common medical treatments for pain. However, you may benefit from reading this section, as you may be unaware of some of the new developments, such as the use of antidepressants for pain. During the period since this book was published, new drugs, surgical procedures, and complimentary modalities and techniques may have become available that can be added to this list and others that can be removed.

Perhaps the most common treatment for pain has been and continues to be medication. The issue with prescription and over-the-counter medications for many people is that, like any drug, they can cause side effects that are unpleasant. These include dizziness, constipation, and problems with concentration. Some side effects can even be dangerous.

Many times, side effects are experienced soon after you begin taking medication. Your physician should monitor side effects carefully, and you should let him or her know about any adverse reactions that you experience.

Long-term use of any medication can cause side effects later in the course of treatment. If you have been taking prescribed medication for a while and begin to experience new symptoms, discuss these with your physician. If you are considering stopping medication at any point, be sure to discuss this with your physician as well. With long-term use of medication, your body may become physically dependent on the drug. Your physician will know how to increase, taper, or stop the medication, and can tell you what you may initially experience as your body adjusts to the change. Changing medication should be always be done under the supervision of a physician.

Analgesic Medication

There are two primary classes of "pain killing" medications (analgesics):

- ◆ Nonnarcotic/nonsteroidal anti-inflammatories: Many pain-alleviating treatments in this class can be purchased without a prescription (e.g., aspirin, Advil, Aleve, Bufferin, Motrin, Tylenol). Others require a prescription (e.g., Celebrex™). These drugs tend to target the peripheral nervous system.
- ◆ Narcotic (opioids). These potent short-acting (e.g., codeine, Dilaudid™, Vicodin™, Lortab™, Percodan™, Percocet™) and long-acting (e.g., methadone, Oxycontin™, Duragesic™) drugs require prescription by a physician. These drugs target the central nervous system (i.e., brain and spinal cord).

Antidepressants

Antidepressants are sometimes effective in relieving pain directly, perhaps due to their effects on serotonin and norepinephrine (neurotransmitters). Antidepressants may also help improve sleep. Therefore, they may be used for pain relief even in the absence of depression. Sometimes antidepressants are prescribed if the emotions accompanying pain interfere with the ability to function and the quality of one's own life. Some antidepressants help with anxiety and are less likely than anti-anxiety medications to cause physical dependency when used over an extended period of time.

Whether to reduce pain directly or to help cope with the effects of having a chronic illness, your physician may have prescribed any of the class of drugs labeled antidepressants (e.g., amitriptyline–Elavil™, doxepin–Sinequan™; imipramine–Tofranil™; trazodone–Desyrel™; Prozac™, Zoloft™). The long-term effects of some of the newest antidepressants are unknown (usually these are the newest selective serotonin and norepinephrine reuptake inhibitors [SSNRI] such as venlafaxine–Effexor™ and duloxetine–Cymbalta™), because they have not been on the market long enough for long-term effects to be studied.

Antidepressant medications usually cause few problems, although they too can cause side effects for some people. If you experience side effects that don't remit after a period of a month or so, or if your side effects are serious (e.g., more than dry mouth or drowsiness, or other minor side effects your doctor should tell you about), let him or her know immediately.

In taking these medications, be aware that they usually take from 2 to 4 weeks before they have an effect. As with any drug, there can also be serious side effects. If you are prescribed an antidepressant and have found it not to be helpful over several months, you should discuss this with your physician and possibly discontinue or change the medication under his or her supervision.

Mixed Agent Drugs

There is one medication that does not exactly fit in any of the other categories that is frequently prescribed for pain—tramadol (Ultram™). At high doses, tramadol has some of the properties of opioids. If you are taking this prescribed medication for your pain and have any problems, you should discuss this with your physician.

Sedatives, Tranquilizers, and Muscle Relaxants

Sedatives and minor tranquilizers (e.g., benzodiazepines)—such as diazepam (Valium™), lorazepam (Ativan™), and clonazepam (Klonopin™)—and muscle relaxants (e.g., cyclobenzaprine–Flexeril™, methocarbamol–Robaxin™), may be prescribed to help people cope with anxiety and also to improve their sleep. These may be used in combination with analgesics. Sedatives and tranquilizers may help relieve short-term anxiety about pain. They also have more immediate effects than antidepressants. However, they are not appropriate for long-term use for people with chronic pain because of their definite potential for addiction when used on a long-term basis (i.e., more than a few months). Again, if you are prescribed any of these medications and have found them not to be helpful after several weeks, you should discuss this with your physician and possibly discontinue or change the medication under his or her supervision.

Anticonvulsants

Anticonvulsant drugs formerly were used only when people had seizures. Now, some anticonvulsants such as gabapentrin (Neurontin™) or topimax (Trileptal™) have been shown to have a beneficial effect on pain associated with nerve injuries for *some* people (e.g., those with diabetic neuropathy, trigeminal neuralgia, postherpetic neuralgia). The long-term effects of these new anticonvulsants are unknown, because they have not been on the market long enough for such effects to be studied.

If you are prescribed any of these medications and have found them not to be helpful in a month or so, you should discuss this with your physician and possibly discontinue or change the medication under supervision.

Topical Agents

Several topical agents, such as (Zostrix™) and 5% lidocaine patch (Lidoderm™) have been shown to reduce the severity of pain in some conditions related to nerve damage. If you are prescribed any of these medications and have found them not to be helpful after several weeks, you should discuss this with your physician and possibly discontinue or change the medication under supervision.

Surgery

Surgery is appropriate with certain kinds of pathology causing acute pain. There are a large variety of surgical approaches that can help, depending on the pathology that is believed to be the "pain generator." However, when pain persists over long periods of time, surgery is less likely to be effective. Also, if you have already had one operation, it is unlikely that more surgery will eliminate the pain. A second operation may, however, be justified if the initial cause of your pain has progressed as part of a degenerative disease, or your physical condition has deteriorated.

When surgery is being considered, you should discuss this with your primary physician and a qualified surgeon. Obtaining a second surgical opinion is recommended, because surgeons differ in their approach to surgery as well. A second opinion also has the benefit of helping you to judge which surgeon is more qualified to conduct the surgery. Because surgery has the potential for ill as well as good, do your homework and be well informed before you elect surgery or choose a surgeon.

Nerve Blocks

Local anesthetic agents (e.g., lidocaine) that are similar to Novocain may be injected into peripheral nerve fibers when the physician believes the pain is being generated, transferred, or referred. The most common form of this procedure is called an *epidural block*. Here, local anesthetic is injected between the vertebrae into spinal nerves. Many other nerves can also be "blocked" by injecting the anesthetic into them. Injection of steroids into the epidural space surrounding the spinal cord and nerves may be helpful in sciatica (leg pain secondary to disc disease). These injections will cause the nerve fibers to become numb (anesthetized). Specially trained physicians, usually anesthesiologists, are qualified to perform nerve blocks.

Some people feel immediate reductions of pain following these injections. Others do not feel any relief. The duration of relief, when obtained, varies unpredictably from hours to days to weeks. However, the effects do not last indefinitely for anyone.

Trigger Point Injections

Trigger points are hypersensitive areas of muscles, ligaments, or tendons. They are known to lie above or near the point in the muscles where the motor nerves are located. Excessive activity in motor nerves can produce pain either at the site or at some other site (i.e., referred pain). There are standard patterns of referred pain associated with specific injuries. When these trigger points are pressed, this can cause a great deal of pain.

Direct stress to the muscle, such as trauma (e.g., a muscle tear during a motor vehicle accident, a tendon inflamed during repetitive activity), chronic tension, abnormal posture, or prolonged muscle fatigue may result in pain in these trigger point areas.

This is relevant to chronic pain, because some who experience chronic pain tend to tense their muscles in an attempt to brace (i.e., protect) them from pain. This, in turn, can lead to the pain–muscle spasm–pain circle. When in spasm, muscles tend to remain in a tense or contracted state, blood flow is decreased to the muscle, and posture can become abnormal. This may serve to maintain the pain or make it worse. Also, some trigger points may become inactive from sedentary living, which is unfortunately common in many chronic pain sufferers. Trigger-point pain can then be reactivated by minor stress from daily living, anxiety, over-stretching, or sudden use, overuse, and fatigue of previously underworked muscles.

Thermal Therapies

Both heat and cold therapy can reduce muscle tension or spasm. Heat can reduce muscle contraction (spasm) caused by overfatigue of muscles. Applying heat to sore, fatigued muscles tends to open (i.e., dilate) blood vessels and thus increase oxygen flow and eliminate chemical irritants. Cold can also reduce muscle spasm and swelling from an injury or inflammation. (Note that many have found that frozen peas in a bag wrapped in a towel are more useful and convenient than ice packs. They can be "molded" around a painful body part such as the forearm. They can be refrozen and used over and over again [be sure not to eat them, afterwards, however]). Heat and cold have been found to be about equally effective and may be used separately or together (i.e., one following the other). They are useful home remedies that are also used during and after physical therapy sessions.

Electrical and Ultrasound Stimulation

Transcutaneous electrical nerve stimulation (TENS) is designed to stimulate nerves to counter-stimulate pain signals (*transcutaneous* means "through the skin"). TENS transmits electrical impulses through wires to surface electrodes taped to the skin surrounding a painful area. The person who is using TENS will feel a tingling sensation that may mask pain signals. TENS may also stimulate the body's own natural pain-reducing chemicals (endorphins—Latin for "internal opioids").

Spinal cord stimulators may be surgically implanted with an external power source. This can be activated to provide an electrical current to nerves along the spinal cord. The electrical current blocks the transmission of signals along the spinal cord so that they do not reach the brain areas that make one aware of pain. Ultrasound, either with heat (in fatty areas) or without heat (in bony areas) has also been found to be useful, particularly in cases of acute injury leading to chronic pain.

Chiropractic Manipulations

In chiropractic theory, muscle and joint pain result from faulty relationships among bones and faulty alignment of the spine. So, chiropractors perform manipulations—often quite strenuously—to return the bones or spinal cord to "proper" alignment. Sometimes these are quite helpful, particularly in the early stages of an injury, such as whiplash. However, over a long period of time they may become less effective.

Acupuncture

Acupuncture is a method of pain and disease control discovered in China almost 5,000 years ago. In acupuncture theory, imaginary lines on the body (called "medians") represent internal organs and other parts of the body. Points on these lines are thought to connect different parts of the body. One or more of these points are stimulated by insertion of an acupuncture needle. When the needles are placed in the skin, the practitioner may gently twirl the needle by hand or by electrical current attached to the needles. Some needles are stimulated for brief periods of 10 to 20 minutes and then removed; others are left in for longer periods of time. The needles used are very thin and solid, and virtually no pain is felt when administered by a qualified practitioner. Currently, the U.S. National Institutes of Health are studying the effectiveness of this treatment for various conditions. As with any treatment, if you decide to have acupuncture, be sure to seek a qualified practitioner.

Biofeedback

Biofeedback is a means of bodily self-monitoring and can be used to help people learn to control certain physiological processes, such as heart rate and muscle tension. For example, under stress, skeletal muscles may contract, causing muscle tension. Biofeedback uses electrical sensors on skin over muscles to detect this rising tension. The electrical sensors are linked to the biofeedback machine, which provides audible or visual signals to the patient. These signals enable people to understand their physiological activities and to control them consciously and, over time, more automatically. With experience, people can determine what mental or physical adjustments produce the greatest reduction in tension. They may then use these exercises without the need of the biofeedback machine. Biofeedback has been used to treat headaches, facial pain (e.g., temporomandibular joint pain), back pain, and fibromyalgia, among other conditions.

Pain Clinics and Rehabilitation Programs

Specialized pain clinics and rehabilitation programs have been developed over the past 30 years to treat people with chronic pain. These programs usually use many of the techniques described above, most often in combination. In addition to including physicians on their staff, the best programs have psychologists specializing in pain reduction who can teach stress management and coping skills. They can also help people improve their communication with family members and health care professionals. The better clinics have physical and occupational therapists on staff to help people learn new ways to improve their strength, endurance, and functioning while they perform household and on-the-job tasks.

Comprehensive programs have been shown to be very effective for helping people with severe, long-standing pain problems. You should discuss the appropriateness of referral to a pain clinic with your primary care doctor. If your doctor is unfamiliar with such clinics, seek out a doctor who is familiar with them (but is not on their staff) and ask whether he or she thinks it is worth your while to try such a program.

Regardless of whether you are taking medication, decide to have surgery, or use any other treatments, be aware that any treatment may reduce but rarely completely eliminates pain for those who experience chronic pain. Thus, the techniques and methods described in this book can be critical in combination with other pain treatments in improving the quality of your life and decreasing pain severity. Also, as mentioned before, some of the treatments just discussed that are useful for some can be completely ineffective for others. If this is your case, then following the lessons in this program is even more crucial. *Anyone* with chronic pain, regardless of the treatment being received, can be helped by following this program.

The Purpose of This Program

When you have chronic pain, life seems to have lost its purpose. Being advised that "you must learn to live with your pain" feels like a betrayal. It is only when you can give purpose and quality to your life that there is a chance you can not only live with the pain, but actually thrive, despite the pain.

With this lesson, you have begun the journey toward a new life by becoming better informed about pain. With knowledge and, most important, application of this knowledge, you will find ways to manage your pain and enjoy your life again.

In the next lesson, the application of knowledge begins. You will learn how to use one of the most important tools in managing your pain—pacing. This next lesson is so vitally important that without it, the remainder of the lessons will likely bring limited relief.

But before ending this lesson, let's recap the high points:

◆ Contrary to what most people think, pain is not always a reliable signal.
◆ You have a right to feel what you feel about your pain. Fear, sadness, frustration, and anger are common responses to feeling helpless about your pain.
◆ The Gate Control Model of pain helps explain some of what is puzzling about pain. There is a pain gate that determines in part whether signals communicating pain reach the brain. Thoughts, feelings, and other factors can open or close the pain gate. In this book you will learn ways to help close the gate.

◆ There are a number of other myths about chronic pain that can be harmful. If you have believed these myths in the past, try to let go of them.

◆ Pain always has something meaningful to say, and for this reason, it should always be taken seriously.

◆ Feelings such as fear, sadness, and anger that often accompany chronic pain can get out of control. Ignoring or denying that you experience these emotions do not help.

Finally, we stress that it's more important to look for the solution than the cause of your pain:

◆ The question is **not** "how did I get the pain?"

◆ The question **is** "how do I manage the pain?"

◆ The question is **not** "what is the cause of the pain?"

◆ The question **is** "what factors influence the pain?"

◆ The question is **not** "what can the medical profession do?"

◆ The question is "what can **I** do?"

In answer to this last question, we have suggested that *you learn to become your own pain management expert.* You know your pain best, and you will be able to design the best pain management program for yourself. We will help you do that in the nine lessons that follow.

The Importance of Action

Remember, knowledge is power. That is why, in part, you are reading this book. But reading is not enough. You must put into action what you learn in each lesson. At the end of this lesson and in all of the following lessons, we raise important questions for you to consider and suggest activities that are critical for pain management. These critical "homework assignments" (i.e., suggested activities) are indicated in boldface type. We have at times suggested additional ones, and doing these can hasten your adjustment. At a minimum, do the critical activities. If you can, do at least one more activity, either the one that appeals to you most or the one that appeals to you least. If you are in a good mood, we suggest that you do the one that appeals to you least. For some reason, these avoided activities can sometimes help the most. Because most people have negative associations to the word "homework," we will call them activities that can help.

Activities That Can Help

To begin, we suggest four activities. Two of these are most important: They involve documenting and rating your recent pain. These are critical because they begin to put on paper a beginning knowledge of your pain that you can build on as you work through this book. Later, as you work through the book, answering these questions can help in reviewing your progress. The other two activities are optional but will definitely help you to become your own pain expert!

Critical Activities

1. Rating your recent pain level. We suggest that you photocopy the Pain Rating System for use now, in the middle of the program, and at the end of the program. You may want to make extra copies for the maintenance phase as well. If you don't have access to a copy machine, use the instructions in parentheses to mark your answers in your notebook or journal.

In considering the ratings, think of each on a continuum. For example, with regard to rating pain, (0) means that you *do not feel even a hint of discomfort. Very intense pain* (6) means that you can barely move without feeling you may pass out from the pain. In the middle (2–5), you are aware of varying degrees of pain. As another example, if you were rating "days," when you are experiencing a (1) level, you are having a *really "good" day.* When you are experiencing a (6) level, you are likely having a *really "bad" day.* In the middle (2–5), you are having a kind of "middle good" or "middle bad" day.

PAIN RATING SYSTEM

1. Rate the level of your pain at the **PRESENT MOMENT**: (Date and record your answer in your journal [i.e., date, intensity].)

| 0 | 1 | 2 | 3 | 4 | 5 | 6 |

No pain   Very intense pain

2. In general, during the **PAST WEEK** how much did your pain interfere with daily activities? (Date and record your answer in your journal [i.e., date, interference].)

| 0 | 1 | 2 | 3 | 4 | 5 | 6 |

No interference   Extreme interference

3. During the **PAST WEEK**, how much has your pain changed the amount of satisfaction or enjoyment you get from taking part in social and recreational activities? (Date and record your answer in your journal [i.e., date, satisfaction change because of pain].)

| 0 | 1 | 2 | 3 | 4 | 5 | 6 |

No change   Extreme change

4. On average, how severe has your pain been during the **PAST WEEK**? (Date and record your answer in your journal [i.e., date, pain severity].)

| 0 | 1 | 2 | 3 | 4 | 5 | 6 |

Not severe   Extremely severe

5. During the **PAST WEEK**, how irritable have you been? (Date and record your answer in your journal [i.e., date, irritability].)

| 0 | 1 | 2 | 3 | 4 | 5 | 6 |

Not irritable   Extremely irritable

6. During the **PAST WEEK**, how tense or discouraged have you felt as a result of your pain? (Date and record your answer in your journal [i.e., date, tension level; discouragement level].)

| 0 | 1 | 2 | 3 | 4 | 5 | 6 |

Not tense/discouraged   Extremely tense/discouraged

We will ask you to repeat your responses to these questions several times through this book. Toward the middle and at the end of the program, you will be able to see how much progress you have made. So, please do your best to respond to each question. However, we ask that you not look back at these ratings until we ask you to do so.

2. Functional pain history

A. Below is a list of activities. Circle the letter of any one that you feel you **can no longer do** because of your pain. (Date and copy these in your notebook or journal.)

a) Cook meals
b) Work on the car
c) Go to the movies
d) Work in the garden
e) Visit with friends
f) Go hunting or fishing
g) Play cards or board games
h) Go to a place of worship
i) Go to/shop at the mall

j) Play sports (golf, tennis)
k) Clean the house
l) Work on hobbies
m) Walk in the park
n) Hold a job
o) Other _____
p) Other _____
q) Other _____

B. Make a list of the things you **CAN** do despite your pain (e.g., talk on the telephone, watch television, read a magazine). (Date and copy these in your notebook or journal.)

C. Circle the letter of the things that have made your pain worse in the past. (Date and copy these in your notebook or journal.)

a) Weather
b) Exercise
c) Stress
d) Cold
e) Heat

f) Arguments
g) Fatigue
h) Poor sleep
i) Depression
j) Other (describe) _____

D. Circle the letter of the things that have made your pain better in the past. (Date and copy these in your notebook or journal.)

a) Rest
b) Warm bath
c) Relaxation
d) Sleep
e) Medication
f) Exercise

g) Other
   (describe) _____
h) Other
   (describe) _____
i) Other
   (describe) _____

Optional Activities

3. Recent pain memories. In your journal or notebook, answer all of the following questions:

  A. Can you remember any day or time when your pain was most intense? In general, what times of day do you feel your pain most?
  B. Were there any activities that tended to increase your pain? What were they?
  C. Were there any stressors that tended to go along with increased pain? What were they?
  D. How did you feel emotionally?
  E. What were you were thinking at the time?
  F. What kinds of behaviors or interactions with others followed the "increased" or intense pain episodes?

4. Describe your pain history as if you were talking to a trusted friend (write this out in your notebook or journal). How long have you had the pain? Where is it located? How has it changed over time? How has the pain affected your work, play, and enjoyment of life? How has the pain affected your relationships with family and friends?

Activity, Rest, and Pacing

Remind me each day
That the race is not always to the swift;
That there is more to life than increasing its speed.
Let me look upward into the towering oak
And know that it grew great and strong
Because it grew slowly and well.
—Orin L. Crain

One of the most frustrating things about pain is that it interferes with your ability to do the things that you want to do. All of the roles you play—parent, partner, breadwinner, friend, neighbor, employee, artist, crafter, gardener, or volunteer—may have been affected. You may feel that you are on the sidelines of life or that life is passing you by.

You may also feel that you are a burden on others when you can't do what you used to do or have to ask for help. You always wanted a meaningful and purposeful life. Now, in your darkest moments, you may wonder if you want a life at all. On better days, you ask yourself "How can I get rid of the pain so that I can get on with my life?" But you feel stuck. You may believe that you have tried everything. You may have actually tried everything doctors have suggested. So, you think to yourself, "I have done what the doctors and other specialists have told me. Why am I still in such pain?"

Or, you may have gotten contradictory advice and don't know which advice to heed. One health care professional may have suggested, "You should take things more easily, you are doing too much." Another, however, suggests, "You should keep moving, you aren't doing enough."

And then there are well-meaning friends and family. You spouse may have told you, "You should persevere, you shouldn't allow yourself to be controlled by the pain." Then, a friend tells you, "You should listen to your body." Not much later, your son calls long distance and tells you, "Don't go by how you feel, push through it." Whose advice are you supposed to follow?

If the advice of others has stymied you, you are not alone. What you really need to do is experiment with your body and become your own expert on what and how much activity really helps. In this lesson, we will help you learn to do that. You will learn to differentiate between the sense and nonsense that others may have suggested.

Knowing what to do about chronic pain is difficult because of its confusing nature. If you have gone to a yoga class or stretching class for "normal" people, the teacher may wisely tell the class, "if you feel pain when you do any of the poses, stop." However, with chronic pain, pain cannot be your only guide with regard to most activities.

Chronic pain may always be present, as you know, but you may have also noticed that it varies in intensity or comes and goes in an unpredictable manner. We will help you learn to deal with this variability and find out what level and type of activity will be most successful for you. You will also learn about the importance of pacing, and that despite some temporary discomfort, you can become active in ways that increase your energy and improve your conditioning.

As you go along, it will become clearer to you how you can regain a level of daily functioning you thought you'd never reach. You may even become more able to do some things than you ever were.

You will learn not only what you can do but also how you can do it better, longer, more efficiently, and without harming yourself or increasing your pain. Yes, we are talking in part about exercise, but don't skip to the next lesson or close the book. If the word "exercise" has always turned you off, think of it as movement. As the saying goes . . .

Move It or Lose It!

How long have you experienced pain? Months, years, decades? Have you tried to prevent pain or at least decrease it by doing less? If so, you may have temporarily reduced your pain, but you may not know the cost of this short-term remedy.

By moving less, you have reduced strength in your muscles. This is because lack of movement immobilizes your muscles, weakens them, and over time increases disability. Over a few months of decreased movement, more activities will become difficult and will begin to cause pain. This additional pain is likely not related to the original cause of pain but to weakened muscles (see Figure 2.1).

This may not make sense to you now. You have learned through experience that certain movements will increase your pain. So, you stop doing them. This appears to be a rational strategy. You know that rest is a necessary condition for healing and recovery. So, you rest. Again, this appears to be a rational strategy.

Well, in one sense it is. In cases of acute pain following an obvious injury, a brief period of rest (several days at most) in the form of inactivity may be useful. But even in these cases, inactivity for more than a week will lead to weakened muscles and increased disability.

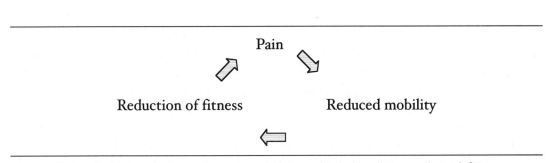

Figure 2.1. Pain leads to reduced mobility, which leads to reduced fitness.

For example, have you ever had a broken arm or leg, or do you know someone who has? Well, if you have, you know that after resetting the bone, a cast is usually placed on the limb to keep it from moving in ways that will increase the injury. This lets the broken bone heal. However, this necessary remedy not only keeps the bone from moving. It also keeps related muscles immobile. When the cast is removed, usually in about 6 weeks, the limb has changed. Comparing that arm or leg with the other that was not injured is clear proof that inactivity causes muscle loss and muscle loss can increase pain.

Studies have shown that we lose 20% of muscle mass, and hence strength, each week that we fail to make use of our muscles! And, if you do not use your muscles there will be a reduction not only in muscle strength but also in flexibility and endurance.

You may be leery of where we seem to be headed. Instead of resting, you may have done the opposite at times—pushed yourself hard, following the Nike command to "Just do it!" But then you have felt much worse for days after. Try to suspend judgment for a time, however, when it comes to this lesson. Try to trust that we're not headed in that direction at all.

Now, being open-minded, you are considering that maybe rest is not always best for healing, and at times it can make things even worse. Perhaps then you will also consider that nongraded activity (i.e., activity that does not build up gradually over time) can cause increased disability. So, what are you to do?

The answer is "balance"—that golden middle that most of us swing through when we go from one extreme to another. When the balance between what you can do and what you actually do is disturbed too often, your body protests, rightfully. The more this signal is ignored the more urgent and louder the protest becomes.

Balance is very personal. What is balance for one person is overwork or underwork for another. So, we need to help you find your personal balance—the amount of movement that does not cause increased chronic pain or increased disability.

We are not saying that this movement won't cause discomfort, especially at first. But discomfort is different from pain. When you suffer chronic pain, it may be difficult to differentiate discomfort from pain, but gradually you will learn how.

The action part of this lesson really begins by asking you to change the way you approach your pain. Are you willing to change your relationship with your body from that of enemies to that of allies?

To achieve this, you may have to change from "always doing it yourself" to asking others to help. You may have to change your style from rigid to flexible. You may have to change the way you solve problems. Or, you may have to do things yourself that you have been asking others to do for you.

You will have to put your health and well-being above other priorities. But we promise that the results will be worth it.

Note that we are not saying that it will always be easy. However, admitting something is difficult when it is in fact difficult can actually be helpful. Telling yourself "this should be easy" when it is hard can make things seem even more difficult. If doing what we advise is hard, let yourself know that it is hard, but persevere.

All real change is difficult, especially change that requires persistence over time. Many people can lose weight, for example. The difficulty comes in maintaining that loss. The same is true with changes in activity levels. The first week you increase your level of activity may seem "not so bad." But, after the novelty wears off, the difficulty may be felt acutely. It's okay to admit this. The key is to persevere despite discomfort.

What about the week you have a fight with your spouse or the day your car doesn't start? Change is hard enough when things are going well, but it becomes even more difficult when things go wrong. Perhaps in these situations you give yourself some slack for a day or so, but no more than that. Again, the key is to persevere.

Move Smarter, Not Harder

One thing has likely become clear to you over time—if you had been able to get better by doing your best, you would have been better a long time ago. This is true even when you have persisted, because when something does not work, the natural tendency is give up or TRY HARDER.

In this lesson, we ask you to list the movement-oriented activities that you have done and ask yourself, "Why didn't it work?" For example, "Could I have tried too hard? Could I have not tried hard enough? Did I not understand or have all the information I needed to do what I had to do (even simple movements or exercises require a learning curve)? Did a life event or stressor interfere with my plan?" This self-knowledge is important, as it will help you to work with us in altering your plan or approach.

In this lesson, we will follow Terry, one of our patients, who suffered from chronic bursitis in her hips (along with other joint problems).

Before Terry worked with us, she felt discouraged. All the remedies suggested by her family doctor failed to bring much relief. She went to a physical therapist for a few sessions, but the exercises she suggested felt boring, and Terry failed to do them regularly. The therapist finally advised that Terry get involved in water exercise or walking, suggesting a few books that Terry patiently wrote down but had no intention of reading. After that session, Terry stopped seeing the physical therapist. But she did decide to try her last suggestion.

Water sounded more interesting than walking, but Terry didn't want to have to get up and get dressed, go to the nearest indoor pool, get wet, and then leave in the cold. A walk sounded really boring. After all, what could walking really do?

Over the December holidays, her 80-year-old father-in-law, Bud, visited their home. Terry and her husband had given him the trip as a holiday present as Bud had never visited their new home.

Although 20 years older than Terry, Bud walked 2 miles in 30 minutes every single day. He was not a braggart, and before his visit Terry never knew that he had a walking regimen. While visiting their home, he took his daily walks. He explained to Terry that he always walked two miles a day and paced himself to be finished in 30 minutes. In the winter and in the heat of the summer, he mall-walked, but in good weather he preferred being outdoors. In Terry's area, they were having a mild winter, so Bud walked outside during his visit.

Terry was impressed. If he could do it, she thought, being so much older than she, she could do it too. After Bud left, she bought a good pair of running shoes (running shoes are suggested for walkers because of the cushioning they provide). Then she marked out a 2-mile path around their neighborhood. She set her goal (Bud's regimen), looked at her watch, and walked the 2 miles in just over 35 minutes. She felt great. The next morning, however, she woke up with tremendous pain in her hips, and stayed in bed for 3 days afterwards. She felt completely hopeless. (To be continued.)

Terry took only age into account. Because the physical therapist, whom she no longer saw, had once suggested walking, she didn't think it could do any harm. Much later, after consulting us, she realized that she had tried to do too much too soon. But Terry's journey didn't stop before she saw us. She kept the water workout in the back of her mind.

The Negative Effects of Others' Responses

Perhaps people close to you (e.g., family, friends) were concerned or less than supportive when they did not see the improvements that they expected when you previously tried to increase your activity level. Perhaps they began to exert pressure on you, which is not very helpful. They may be well meaning, but they are typically not people who suffer from chronic pain themselves. They don't know that you typically put yourself under enough pressure as it is.

For the time being, it is best to start your new level of activity in a quiet way. Don't tell anyone who is apt to have too-high expectations that you are beginning a new program. It is more important in the beginning that you learn to enjoy movement once again than for you to chance a nonsupportive "support network." Of course, once you start "exercising" to any extent, you will want to discuss details of your exercise program with your physician or physical therapist. As mentioned in the beginning of this book, our advice is not a substitute for the advice of your physician.

First Steps to Enjoying Activity

The first step in making activity or movement enjoyable is a mental step. You will need to work on changing the way you conceive of activity by thinking of it as a "want" or "choice" rather than a "must" or "should." You may not think that such wording makes a difference. But listen to how it feels when you say to yourself "I get to do this" rather than "I must do this." Try talking to yourself this way for a month and see what a difference it makes in your attitude, not just about activity, but about life in general. Choosing to do something rather than pressuring yourself to do it will reduce stress. Because stress increases one's awareness of pain, decreased stress will in turn decrease your awareness of pain.

Second, you'll benefit by changing the way you view "good days" and "bad days," which people with chronic pain frequently have. Why do we suggest this? If you have had good days and bad days, you may have found that on the good days you try to catch up on what you feel you have neglected on the bad days. So, you push yourself on the good days only to find that you are exhausted and unable to do much of anything on the next day. Over time, this pattern of pushing yourself on good days and then being too exhausted to do much of anything on the following days will make your pain worse. You will also find that you have fewer good days and more bad ones if you continue in this way.

Instead of viewing days as good or bad, think of them as "easy" or "challenging." On both kinds of days, try to keep to a regular schedule of activity. We'll have more to say about this later in this lesson. But for now let us reassure you: We know that you can't do the same thing on easy days as on challenging days. Later, we will describe how on challenging days you will still stay active, but you might have shorter periods of exertion followed by longer periods of rest and recuperation.

The challenge here is to pace yourself, maintaining a reasonable, consistent schedule of activity. Sure, you may do somewhat less on the good days and the bad days at first, but by pacing yourself you will be able to accomplish more than you did when you pushed yourself too hard on one day and then were laid up afterwards. More important, by not overexerting yourself on the good days, you will be able to have a greater number of days when you feel better (note that we did not say totally pain free).

The third step is to think of movement as something you will increase gradually. You want to move from Pattern A to Pattern B and finally to Pattern C, as shown here. Here you can see the gradual change in the activity–rest cycle. In Pattern A, a little activity is followed by a long period of rest. How to achieve this change is what this lesson is all about.

Pattern A

Activity	Rest	Activity	Rest	Activity	Rest

After a few weeks of pacing, you will be in somewhat better shape. Then, your pattern may be like Pattern B, when the periods of rest and activity are more in balance.

Pattern B

Activity	Rest	Activity	Rest	Activity	Rest

After continued pacing and gradually increasing, your activity level you will achieve a more optimal balance of activity and rest, as shown in Pattern C.

Pattern C

Activity	Rest	Activity	Rest	Activity	Rest

Many people set a kitchen timer or pay attention to their watch on their good days, so that they won't unintentionally overdo. People who work at computers all day have used the same trick to remind them to stretch or walk around every 20 minutes or so. Working at a computer without frequent stretching can lead to chronic pain problems (e.g., in the shoulders and back).

Like yo-yo dieting, which has been shown to be harmful, yo-yo active–passive days are bad for your health as well. The important thing is to find the right balance between doing too little and too much. Before we tackle the most important tool in achieving balance–pacing, let's return to Terry to see what **not** to do in achieving balance.

Terry needed more physical therapy after she overdid it walking. The therapist again suggested gentle water walking. So, Terry decided to look into water exercise courses available in her community. She finally found a drop-in class geared for seniors (i.e., those over 55), so she thought this would work. Without checking with her doctor or physical therapist, she bought a cheap pair of water walking shoes and signed up for the class.

The first class she attended on Monday was great. The teacher had arranged for the water to be warm, and Terry found that getting dressed and going out actually didn't feel so bad. That night, she slept soundly for the first time in months. Part of the fatigue was due to learning the new movements in class, but part of it was getting out and moving again.

The second class was on Wednesday. This time, Terry was familiar with the moves, so she could focus more on working hard like the others in the class. She couldn't keep pace with them yet, but she tried to do her best. She assumed she would be at their level soon.

Terry rested until the next class on Monday. This time, she was determined to keep up with the class. After all, water would cushion her joints (or so a magazine article said), and she reminded herself that there were people much older than she in the class.

The following day she felt as bad physically as she had felt after her first 35-minute walk. Emotionally, she felt even worse. Terry felt she had "failed" again. (To be continued.)

Terry forgot that, as with the walking, age is not the only factor to take into account when signing up for a class. Is the class geared to beginners? That is an important consideration. Is the teacher credentialed? Has he or she worked with individuals with injuries or chronic pain?

Terry's class had students of all levels. Terry's teacher had worked with seniors, and had excellent water aerobic training, but she was new and had no experience with rehabilitative water work.

Terry was also unaware that as we grow older, particularly when we have chronic pain or injuries, the time between strenous classes may need to be differently scheduled. Monday and Thursday, rather than Monday and Wednesday, would have been better for Terry. Finally, Terry didn't realize that a class can, even if one is not competitive, bring out the need to keep pace with others. So, let's carefully examine now what Terry would later learn— the steps involved in pacing.

How to Pace Yourself

Pacing involves several steps that we will describe in detail later in this section. First, though, an overview. The initial step in pacing is to select an activity that you would like to do or would like to do more of. The second is to develop a baseline (i.e., where you are now with regard to that activity). The third is to set short-term goals and assess progress. And the fourth is to set longer term goals and continue the assessment process.

Selecting Your First Activity

Begin with just one activity (later you can add more). This can be a chore, or it can be a hobby or a form of exercise. Perhaps you would like to do more housework than you are currently doing. For some people, an orderly house is a real stress-reducer.

Perhaps you would like to play golf longer or walk more during your game (i.e., ride around in the golf cart less). Perhaps you would like to do volunteer work in a community agency. If you have children at home, perhaps you would like to be more involved in their activities.

Selecting the right first activity is important. You want it to be something that is realistic to do and motivating as well. If you choose something too hard, you will feel discouraged. If you choose something distasteful (e.g., doing more cooking when you didn't like to cook even when you were well), you will not have an experience that you will look forward to. Later on, you can take on tasks that don't appeal to you but need doing nonetheless. But first, choose something realistic and motivating.

It doesn't have to be big or dramatic. Perhaps you have been bed-bound. An increase in activity may simply be getting up and walking around the bed one time. Perhaps you only move from one chair to the sofa to a table and to bed. An increase in activity would be walking around the room several times. Someone with serious back problems should not carry large weights, but making the bed may be an achievable goal. Someone with shoulder tendon problems should not lift large numbers of plates at a time, but unloading the dishes one by one from the dishwasher for 5 or 10 minutes can help.

This is nothing, you may think. How am I ever going to accomplish anything at this pace? Please don't think that these small activities will not eventually lead to something more exciting. Trust us, they will. What you are doing in the beginning is getting a taste for success and gradually building stamina.

If you are more mobile currently, you may want to consider exercising. If you have not exercised for a long time, it is likely that few forms of exercise will be appealing. Our advice here is to choose the one that is simplest and that you dislike least.

Here are a few forms of exercise that our patients have found least objectionable when they first started exercising: walking on a treadmill or other flat surface while listening to music, swimming at a very leisurely pace, doing gentle stretching exercises, working with small hand-held weights (e.g., 1–2 pounds). For our patients with joint or back pain, simply walking in water at an indoor pool (at a depth that is about the same height as your chest) has been particularly helpful.

Some of our patients have found gentle yoga or one-on-one pilates (the latter of which was originally developed for rehabilitation) to be useful. However, be sure that you know the qualifications of the instructor, as yoga and pilates can cause serious injury if not done properly and under adequate supervision. Also, we recommend that you don't take these classes at a regular fitness center or club, because those kinds of places tend to group people together at differing ability levels. Beginners almost always overexert themselves without meaning to. A specialized yoga or pilates studio is best.

However, if you tend to be competitive, it is best to stay away from any type of group activities for a while (e.g., a water aerobics class). Once you know your baseline (i.e., the next step you will learn) in a particular area, you can begin to compete (slowly!) with yourself.

Chances are greater that you will not overextend yourself when you have set reasonable goals for yourself than if you try to keep up or compete (even unknowingly) with others. On the other hand, if you have an activity buddy with the same level of endurance and speed, then this can make some activities (such as water walking) more pleasurable. You can also encourage each other on days when you don't feel like moving. But if someone else's endurance or speed is above your level, you can fall into the same trap of trying to keep up with a friend that you would in a group activity.

Think about the exercises we have discussed, and others that you may think of. Keep in mind that almost any form of movement that is not contraindicated by your physician will be helpful if you do it gradually. However, whereas exercise is one of the best ways to build stamina, it is not necessary to choose exercise in the beginning. It is most important to choose an activity that you can and will do, and that you find appealing and motivating.

Developing Your Baseline

The second step in pacing is deciding on a a reasonable amount of time to spend during your first week of increased activity or on how much exercise you will try to do (e.g., distance walked, number of repetitions). To do this, you must first develop your baseline.

A baseline is simply what you are able to do now in your selected activity. This baseline is the activity level that you will gradually build upon. Most people have no idea of what they can normally do. But determining this baseline is critical in order for you to progress.

To illustrate how developing a baseline works, let's look at weight management programs for a moment. When people embark on a well-designed program, they are often counseled to write down what they normally eat for a week. They are told not to change it, just to record it. (Few people can resist changing their eating patterns after a few days, however.)

You are going to do the same with your chosen activity, but not for a week, just for two days. If you have been doing some of the activity you have chosen already, simply do what you normally do and stop when you normally stop. Write down how you feel emotionally and physically before and after you do the activity. If it is an activity you do daily, we suggest that you record the activity on both a "bad day" and on a "good day." Other than this, please do not do anything different with regard to this activity than you would normally do on these days.

If you are beginning a new activity, do 10% to 20% *less* than you estimate you can do without a significant increase in the amount of pain or fatigue you are now experiencing. For example, if you decide to go for a walk, and you think you can walk 5 minutes, walk only 4. This will help you not overexert yourself in the zeal of getting started. Do this on both a "good day" and on a "bad day." Record in your journal or notebook how you felt before and after, physically and emotionally, on both days.

At first, some of you may only be able to move for a few minutes or do a few repetitions of an exercise (e.g., gently stretching your neck from side to side five times, performing three sit-ups, walking a quarter of a block). This is absolutely fine. The important thing is that you have started!

Setting Short-Term Goals

Weekly Goals

The next step is to set a goal for the activity or exercise for each day of the first week you plan to begin increasing your activity level. Try not to put this off too long. On the other hand, don't start a new activity program during a week that is packed with obligations already. You want to experience success!

The first 2 or 3 days we suggest that you set your goals at your baseline level. This will allow you to monitor how you are doing on consecutive days. We expect that you will feel *some* discomfort. For most people, this discomfort is caused by using muscles that have weakened over time. By increasing your activity level in a reasonable fashion, you are not doing yourself any harm! Over time you will feel less and less discomfort even as you increase your activities.

As recommended earlier, whether you are having a good day or a bad day, try to stick to your initial plan as much as possible. Let your goal of recovery be your guide, not your initial level of discomfort after increasing your activity level.

However, it should be stressed that discomfort and serious increases in pain are not the same thing! Gauge your discomfort each day. If it is minor to moderate, don't worry. If it is significant or if you must rest for an abnormally long time before you recover from the activity, you are likely doing too much and need to cut back.

An important part of beginning to increase your activity level is to pay close attention to the amount of rest you need between activities. Your weekly schedule of activities (which includes your daily schedule) should be a balance of more active and less active days. Your body will rest and rejuvenate during the less active days. Your body will build strength and endurance on the more active days. The key is to not under- or overstress your capacity. This is true for activities in a single day as well.

Let's say you are trying to increase the amount of household chores you are doing. You will need to build in adequate rest time if you plan to do two chores. For example, vacuuming for 15 minutes once in the morning, followed by a half hour break, followed by 15 minutes unloading the dishwasher may be reasonable for you. But doing both activities together (i.e., 30 minutes at a stretch) may cause too much of a strain in the beginning. Eventually you will build up to 30 minutes of housework in one stretch. But it is particularly important not to overdo it in the beginning.

It is also important to keep in mind which basic muscle groups you are working when you are doing more than one activity in a day. Say, for example, you have decided to exercise using light weights. People who lift heavier weights to keep fit are told not to work the same muscle groups two days in a row. Typically, they allow 24 hours before working those muscles again (as they get older, they may need 36–48 hours recovery time).

This is true for light weights as well. Your muscles should feel a tad achy the day after you have worked them; this is normal and a sign that they are becoming stronger. Even if you don't feel achy, you should allow at least 24 hours recovery time before working these muscles again. If you want to do something the next day, do something that works a different set of muscles (e.g., if you lift 1-pound weights one day, perhaps you can walk a block or so [depending on your baseline] on the next day). This allows you to strengthen both your upper-body and lower-body muscles.

On the other hand, you don't want to allow too much rest time between periods or days of being active. Even professional athletes must watch out for this. For example, elite cyclists vary the intensity and type of activities they engage in. When there is a rest day in the Tour de France Bicycle Race, the racers actually continue to exercise, although they might not ride their bikes at all on that day. If the cyclists did not stay active and spent their entire day in bed, the next day their legs would feel like lead, and they would suffer in both body and performance.

The key for you is to find that magic balance between resting too much and resting too little, doing too much and doing too little. What used to be acceptable when you did *not* suffer chronic pain (i.e., clenching your teeth, ignoring the pain, and pushing ahead without rest) will have a negative effect when the pain is chronic. The more you do this, the less you will actually achieve. The same goes for excessive rest.

What happens to people with chronic pain who rest too much between activities? Exactly the same thing as would happen to elite cyclists if they didn't stay active between hard cycling days. The next time they were active they would feel debilatated. "Hold on," you might be thinking, "What is all this talk about elite athletes? I'm not an elite athlete. Never was, and never will be." Well, neither are we. But in the same way that athletes do, we must all learn the proper balance between activity and rest. In short, we must all learn to pace ourselves.

Finally, keep in mind that it is important to increase activities that involve areas of your body where you are not experiencing any pain. Ask yourself, "What parts of my body and what movements cause me the least pain?" When you exercise these areas, it has a positive influence on the rest of your body, including the parts where you most experience pain. Such activities stimulate breathing and the circulation of blood throughout the body. Afterwards, you are better able to relax, and this relaxation enables more energy for the things you enjoy (see next lesson). In short, one part of a reasonable exercise program is to **make the strong body parts stronger.** Indirectly, this will benefit the weaker and painful parts of your body.

Goals for the Month
Goals should be set after the first week so that you are slowly increasing the amount of time you are doing an activity or increasing the number of times that you do it. If you are having problems meeting your initial goals (i.e., excessive pain or fatigue), then cut back and work more slowly. But keep moving ahead.

No two people are the same or change at the same rate, and this makes it particularly important to develop an activity plan that is suited to you personally. You can consult with your doctor or physical therapist if you need more help in developing realistic goals. But remember that only you know if you tend to go at things too hard (and then fizzle out) or whether you're too easy on yourself and are therefore unlikely to achieve much, even over an extended period of time.

If, after increasing an activity (such as a chore or a hobby), you decide to add an exercise program (and we recommend this later), remember to get a baseline, start slowly, and build gradually. If you don't take a daily walk, don't try to cover six blocks your first time out.

Again, if you are the kind of person who tends to go to extremes, be careful not to overdo it, no matter which activities you chose. Don't be afraid of a little discomfort, but don't be reckless either!

If you are progressing very slowly and are still in a lot of pain after exertion, decrease your levels of activity below your initial baseline. Do not immediately conclude, "That is absolutely worthless. I am already doing so little." Remember, we are only on lesson 2. The more impatient you are feeling, the slower you should go in the beginning. Later on, you can push yourself a little harder. But for now, trust our advice.

Progressing Over Time

Once you have some experience with increasing activity levels without undue pain, you can try increasing them at a brisker pace (e.g., increasing the activity 10%–20% [in the case of walking] or by 2–3 minute increments [in terms of other activities]) on a biweekly or weekly basis. However, do not increase at this level if you are doing light weight lifting. Weight lifting requires slower increases in time or in intensity.

In general, remember that the human body is not built to handle extreme changes. For example, if you've ever traveled overseas, you can tell how difficult it is for your body to adjust to the sudden time change. You might also think of someone who is active during the warmer months but becomes a coach potato during the winter. When the first nice day of spring arrives, he spends the day playing golf. The sun feels so good and the movement so natural, he forgets that he is using muscles that haven't been worked for several months.

Each year it comes as a surprise when he feels stiff and achy the following day. Later in the season, he may not feel the same way because the muscles involved in golfing have been strengthened. The same is often true for avid gardeners. The first week of glorious spring can wreak a week of agony for knees and hips. And these are people who do not suffer from chronic pain!

(A note for the eager: Once you have mastered progressing slowly and with consistency, you may be able to increase your activity level every other day. But monitor yourself for signs of overfatigue and pain.)

Assessing Progress Over Time

If you have kept daily records of activities and rest periods, you may find it motivating to see visually how you are progressing over time. Some people find it helpful to keep track of progress using a bar graph or chart (see *Activities That Can Help* at the end of this lesson).

Summary

To recap the most important points in pacing, when increasing activity levels, develop a baseline and build up slowly and with respect for your body. Once you have set your weekly and monthly goals, you should try to stick to them. Do not do more of your activity (even on good days) and do not do less, unless you are having a particularly bad day. Then, decrease by 10% to 20% (or more if necessary), but try not to completely stop being active that day. You want to stay in the optimal level of activity, which means neither overdoing nor underdoing what you are capable of. On that note, let's see how Terry's journey ended.

When Terry consulted us, we explained that her problems with activity were not due to increasing her activity levels but to doing so in an unbalanced way. We agreed with her physical therapist's initial recommendation for walking, but we worked with her to develop a baseline first. We asked her what she thought was a reasonable time or distance she could walk slowly. She thought for a while and then said 15 minutes. Because we could tell she tended to overestimate her readiness, we advised her to try only 10 minutes the first week in establishing her baseline, and monitor herself carefully for an exacerbation of pain. She then asked about two 10-minute walks a day. Again, we told her to start with only one 10-minute walk a day.

Then she asked about adding water aerobics. Couldn't she walk in the morning and do some water exercises in a class in the afternoon? Because she, like many other people, have a hard time not overdoing in a group situation, we ruled those classes out until Terry had more experience getting to know her capabilities and limitations. We also did not want her to experience undue stress in trying NOT to keep up with others at this point. In short, we wanted her to experience success this time! And, you will be happy to know that she did.

How Pain and Inactivity Have Affected You

When people feel pain, it affects their posture—the way they sit, stand, and move. In effect, they unconsciously adapt their posture to the pain.

Pain may also make their movements slower, less coordinated, and erratic (e.g., they may jerk when they don't mean to). They might move in a rigid and protected fashion.

Stop reading for a moment and become aware of how you are sitting. Are you upright? Listing to one side? If you don't notice anything sitting, get up and naturally walk across a room toward a mirror. Was your movement slow, tense, did you feel a tad off balance? Were you stooped in any way? Leaning to one side?

Some people who have back pain, for example, may limp slightly. The intent of limping is to protect from pain, but this distorted movement not only reduces strength in the affected muscles but also places strain on the muscles that have to compensate for the awkward movement. Others who have been involved in a motor vehicle accident may have developed whiplash. To avoid pain, they hold their heads in a rigid way and reduce their neck movements. Over time, people become unaware of the restrictions or the awkwardness of their movements.

They have become **habits.** Restricting or altering correct movement in areas of any chronic pain may reduce pain temporarily but over time will lead to weakened muscles and more pain.

In almost all cases of chronic pain, people contract more muscles than may be necessary even if it does not show in the mirror. These minute corrections have also been a well-intentioned effort to decrease or minimize pain. However, this too leads over time to more pain and greater disability.

Many people with chronic pain become less active over time. One consequence of inactivity is weight gain, especially around the stomach. This added weight coupled with weakened abdominal muscles places a strain on the back and can also cause postural changes that add to pain. Once you decrease activity, over time you will feel increased fatigue, leading to more inactivity, more pain—a viscious revolving door that is difficult to exit.

The question, then, is not whether you should be active. The question is how much activity you should perform, for how long, and in what way. In a nutshell, that is what this lesson has been all about! The goal of this is to improve strength, endurance, and flexibility, which will over time lead to decreased pain. It's best, if you can swing it, to stop reading at this point and actually work on increasing your activity level by pacing. Only by doing, experiencing, and recording the results will you find out where you are now and how quickly in time and intensity you can increase your activity level.

Getting started with an activity plan is critical. Assume that you will need to adjust it as your body gives you feedback (and, again, discomfort is not the same as pain when it comes to bodily feedback).

A Note About Setbacks

When you set up an activity or exercise program, it is likely that you will have setbacks at times (see also lesson 10). It's helpful to know that this is a normal part of the change process. Those on a food plan may follow it rigorously for three weeks and then suddenly eat twice their allotted calories one on day. Falling off and getting back on the horse almost always accompany progress at certain points. Even if you do everything perfectly correctly, sometimes you will experience a spontaneous flare-up of pain. Or, you will have three highly stressful days in a row (especially around the holidays).

Nothing seems to work well when it is an all-or-nothing approach. Pushing yourself with "musts" doesn't work as well as does encouraging yourself to start your day over, even if it is 3 p.m. in the afternoon.

As mentioned in the first part of this lesson, a systematic and gradual expansion of activities may initially cause your experience of pain to increase somewhat as you use unused muscles. Ultimately, however, the discomfort will decrease and the pain will decrease as you strengthen your muscles. For some, even if the overall decrease in pain seems minor over time, you will notice that more has become possible with less effort. And, the more reasonably active you are, the less you will tend to focus on the pain and the more you will enjoy daily life.

The effort and concentration that used to go into protecting yourself might first go into strengthening areas adjacent to the area in which the pain occurs. For example, someone with a weak and painful back needs to begin by strengthening abdominal (stomach), arm, and leg muscles.

Common Problems When Becoming More Active

We know that it is difficult to begin to become more active when you have been immobile for a while. We know that it is difficult to exercise when you experience chronic pain and fatigue. (Even those without chronic pain find getting started in an exercise program difficult!) However, we also know from years of clinical experience that becoming more active in a planned and rational way will increase your strength, endurance, and flexibility, and will ultimately decrease your pain.

Over time, our patients have shared their doubts about this with us, and perhaps you have a few of these doubts as well. We will try to tell you on paper what we tell them face-to-face.

I worry that the exercise will make me feel even worse. Remember, any new activity will temporarily increase discomfort. Work at a level that does not cause excessive pain while doing the exercise and afterwards. Gradually increase your efforts so that overuse or misuse does not result in more pain. If the way you are doing the exercise causes pain or if you really fear that the activity will make you worse, review your activity plan with your doctor or physical therapist.

I've always gotten bored easily doing exercise. Boredom is sometimes a mask for frustration. It takes time to recondition the body, and many people give up before they see improvement. If this is not the case, however, find a more enjoyable environment or activity. Some people do better in *noncompetitive* fitness facilities, a place in which they are surrounded by others. Some do better alone. Set specific reasonable goals each week and each time you exercise. Keep careful track of your activities so that you can see progress in black and white.

I've always relied on my pain to tell me when I'm doing well or poorly. What can I rely on now? Pain is important to monitor when you are exercising or becoming more active in other ways. But it is not a useful guide to determine whether you are doing well. Especially in the beginning, it is better to rely on your level of effort. Later on, it will be better to focus on your ability to move further, easier, or longer as your guide for success.

I always tend to do too much too fast. How can I stop doing this? Doing too much, too fast is a common problem. Start slowly. Begin with easy repetitions with a relaxation pause of 5 to 10 seconds between repetitions. Do not use fast, jerky movements. Do the exercise just hard enough to feel a gentle stretch to the muscles. Do not apply force to the muscle so that you develop increased pain while you are stretching. Remember, building up your flexibility, endurance, and strength is an ongoing and gradual process. Overdoing it one day will interfere with your progress on the next.

In short, make a reasonable plan, keep charts of your daily activity levels and do not give into the temptation to speed up toward your ultimate goal when you are experiencing success.

I don't know how to exercise. Exercise is a learned activity, just like driving a car. You may want to enlist the help of a physical therapist or a certified personal trainer who is experienced with people with disabilities and chronic pain to teach you technique. Such individuals are available in private practice or as part of large public fitness facilities. As you practice, check your technique in front of a mirror periodically. As in golf, good practice makes you better, poor practice makes you worse!

I've tried exercising before, but I always gave up. What's going to be different this time? This time you will prepare yourself mentally to begin, by using all the suggestions made in this lesson. You may need time to experiment, but you will find a program of activity that fits your unique personality and circumstances. And, you will not be alone. We will be on the journey with you.

Activities That Can Help

Critical Activities

Choose an activity you would like to do or to do more of. Follow the instructions for pacing that were detailed in this lesson.

If you haven't started to exercise, after 2 or 3 weeks of increasing your other activities, begin to incorporate exercise into your weekly routine. Follow the guidelines for pacing detailed in this lesson.

Optional Activities

Establish a baseline with regard to your general activity level. How many hours a day do you spend sitting, lying down, standing, and exercising, including doing household chores? This will allow you to later see how much more active you have become on a daily basis.

In the space below record the number of hours you do each of these activities:

Sitting ——————— hours

Lying down ——— hours

Standing ——————— hours

Chores or other activities ——————— hours

Exercise ——————— hours

Sleeping ——————— hours

Total = 24 hours

Construct an activity schedule (i.e., walking, swimming, or cycling). Use the chart as a guide. It can be used for any activity. The numbers along the left can be set for the number of minutes, a distance, or the number of repetitions. Remember to start low, increase slowly, and record your performance each day.

Activity Schedule

Activity: _____

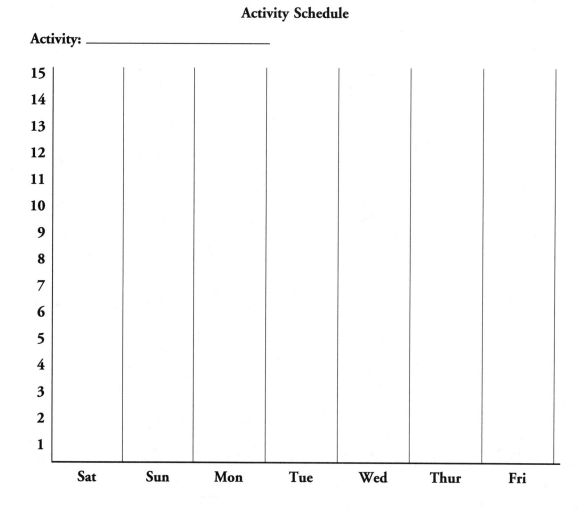

Learning to Relax

All men's miseries derive from not being able to sit quiet in a room alone.
—Blaise Pascal

With continual pain, you may feel that you are waging a battle with your body all day. Pain may feel like the enemy—a monster that that makes you afraid of tomorrow, keeps you from sleeping tonight, and stops you from enjoying today. A result of this battle is that you may feel all kinds of negative emotions that add to your pain.

You want to fight the pain monster or run away from it, but you find that you can't fight and you can't flee. So, you feel demoralized and stuck.

When you try to relax, it feels like a car in neutral gear with someone else stepping on the gas. Your engine revs but you can't move forward. High arousal and tension levels leave you too exhausted to move.

Along with this internal pressure, you may feel pressure from others to be more productive. It may be true that your family, friends, partner, children, doctor, insurance company, and employer are in fact making life more difficult by their lack of understanding. Or, you may be reading things into others' looks or words, but you are so exhausted, you don't realize this. If you are the breadwinner in the family or your own sole support, you may also develop financial problems that add to your distress. If you are the home manager, you may feel guilty that you can no longer do as much. You worry that others are thinking the same thing you worry about much of the time—that you may never get well.

These stressors and others all interfere with your ability to get adequate rest and a good night's sleep. This in turn creates another vicious circle. It is much easier to cope with pain when you are rested, but because you never seem to feel rested anymore, your coping is impaired. This leads to even more problems.

In this lesson you will learn about these and other causes of tension and restlessness. More important, you will learn the positive effect of relaxation on your energy balance and on your experience of pain. Most important, you will learn how to truly relax again—despite your level of pain at the moment.

When you increase your ability to relax and achieve a more restful sleep, you will begin to feel more energetic and you will gain a new sense of control over your life. You will notice that being more relaxed lessens the severity of your pain and decreases the negative effects of pain on your life.

The Energy Balance

In today's fast-paced and overbooked world, it is difficult for most people to maintain the balance between effort and relaxation. We are bombarded every day with seemingly endless amounts of information. And not only is the information highway crowded, actual highways have failed to keep pace with growing populations in many areas. Cell phones have been a wonderful boon in terms of being able to coordinate schedules, contact help when a car breaks down, or let your employer or family know if you're going to be late. But they have had the unintended effect of making people feel that they must always be available.

A minority of families are able to afford for one person to stay at home and keep the household running. But most people need two incomes, especially if they have children to clothe, feed, and educate. Single parents are under tremendous stress. The majority of people try to do too much.

When you add chronic pain to this equation, you can see why you may feel stressed most of the time. To help, well-meaning people tell you that you have to take time for yourself to reduce stress. However, you often find that if you do, you are too exhausted to enjoy it. Shopping is no longer a pleasant pastime, but a tedious hunt—for a parking place, for a bargain, and then for a place to put that bargain.

Without meaning to, most of us get caught up in this hectic pace until our bodies go on strike. We come down with a cold or the flu or we wrench a muscle. People who are living with chronic pain are not immune to further illness or injury.

There is no such thing as a life without tension. But there is an optimal level of stress. Without changes that call for adaptation, life would be boring. But too much stress over too long a period of time is not good for anyone, especially you.

Those who suffer from chronic pain often feel guilty about the idea of relaxing when they are contributing less than they used to. But they are no different in their needs to recharge your batteries and leave the stress behind for a while. In the previous lesson, we emphasized the value of activity. In this lesson, we emphasize the other part of the equation—true rest and relaxation.

Are You Overstressed?

How do you know if you are indeed overstressed? Here are some clues: You want to do many things at the same time; you consistently want to do more than you are capable of;

you want to do nothing at all; you attempt to take control of things that are not in your control (e.g., other people, places, and events).

Stress and these symptoms of stress take energy away from you. Think of energy like you think of money. When the expenses are higher than the income, sooner or later you'll be in financial trouble. When your body uses up more energy than it produces, you will feel physically and emotionally bankrupt.

This may be hard to believe when you think about how you have been doing less and less since your pain began. But living with pain is another stressor unless you learn how to manage the pain through a balance of activity *and* relaxation.

If you are having trouble grasping this, think of it this way. When you are overstressed or underrelaxed, the muscles in your body naturally tense. This means that at least half of your body weight is under tremendous pressure. This pressure can increase your heart rate and cause shallow breathing, which increases fatigue and exhaustion. Furthermore, for many people, proper nutrition is the first thing that is sacrificed when they are under stress. They either eat too much, too little, or the wrong food. In any case, their body is running on the wrong amount or type of fuel. Most important, these effects of being over stressed and under relaxed can increase your pain.

Let's try another analogy, because people are surprisingly resistant to suggestions that they need to relax. When you buy a car, you're interested in whether your car will last over time. You're also interested in whether this complicated machine will need special maintenance. With energy costs skyrocketing, you're most certainly interested in the prospective car's fuel consumption and how this fits in with your budget.

Your body is complex, much more so than your car. If you want your body to have enough fuel to enjoy your life, you have to make it more energy efficient. And you certainly want to conserve fuel so that you can take care of routine activities. This is where relaxation comes in. When your body is tense, your muscles are consuming unnecessary fuel, fuel that you need for enjoyment and for the requirements of daily life.

Conserving Energy

The first step in conserving fuel is to learn to know when you are tense and when you are relaxed. This is more difficult than most people think. Very often, people are unaware of their bodies, except for the experience of pain. Especially when you are under tension for extended periods, you are unconsciously tense and unknowingly consuming a great deal of fuel. Tension is both mental and physical. Let's try a small exercise to help you learn what physical tension feels like.

Make a fist with your right hand. Clench your fist tightly. Really squeeze it tight. Feel your fingers pushing into your palm. Hold it there!

Now bring your clenched fist up toward your shoulder and press the fist against your shoulder. Feel the muscles in your forearm and your biceps (the muscle between your elbow and shoulder) begin to quiver. Hold it there. Count to five.

This is muscle tension. If you keep this up long enough, you will experience pain, eventually even unbearable pain.

Now, compare how your left hand and arm feel in comparison with your right. Note the different feelings and sensations between the right and the left hands and arms. Your left is in a state of relaxation; your right is in a state of tension.

Now, slowly relax your fist and arm. Bring your fist down from your shoulder slowly. Let your muscles relax. Move your fingers away from your palm, relaxing your fist. Slowly bring your fist and arm down to rest loosely on the arm of your chair, a table, or your lap.

Do you see how different this feels? This is relaxation. Relaxation feels different to different people. For some doing this exercise, their right hand feels warm. For others, it tingles, feels a bit heavy, or feels very light.

Notice the difference in how your right hand and arm feel now compared with when you tensed them.

Even with this short exercise, you have learned that you have some control over muscular tension and that you can bring about muscle tension and muscle relaxation through conscious effort to some degree. This means that you have more control over your daily tension levels than you previously thought and that you have power that you have not yet harnessed. In this lesson, we hope to help you learn how to harness this power to reduce your pain.

Sources and Symptoms of Excess Stress

Because excess muscular tension is often unrecognized, it is helpful first to learn more about the most frequently occurring sources and symptoms of chronic muscular tension and stress. Be aware that rarely do people have all these symptoms, and that what is stressful for one person may not be for another.

Here are some of the sources and symptoms people in our practices have shared:

Sensory Overload
Heavy traffic, noisy groups of people, and loud radio and television advertisements make many people tense. Some people with chronic pain report problems with bright lights; others feel greater sensitivity to cold and damp weather.

How about you? Stop and think for a moment. Have you noticed a lower tolerance for some forms of sensory stimulation than you had before your pain began?

Emotional Vulnerability

When people have chronic pain, they commonly feel distressed and overwhelmed, but they often stifle their emotions, especially over small things, until they feel they will explode. Then, they may break down and cry or have a fit of temper at unexpected times. These outbursts are troubling, but it helps to know that they are almost always a result of stored tension.

Some of these negative emotions you feel or stifle are triggered by the sense of futility you have felt over managing your pain. You may then feel guilty about mood changes or "irrational feelings." Guilt alone is a great stressor.

How has your pain influenced your mood? Do you often feel upset, angry, or depressed? Some people have difficulty accepting these negative feelings. It is okay to admit these feelings, if only to yourself.

Such feelings are not unusual, but they can contribute to increased muscle tension and thereby increased pain. People with chronic pain have often adapted to this by tuning out their bodies as much as possible.

The first step in dealing with the stress that is draining your energy is to pay closer attention to your body. By this we mean that the next time you notice a feeling, begin to pay attention to all of your bodily sensations. Do you notice any tension in any of your muscles? Does your body feel numb (except for the pain)? It takes time and practice to tune in to your body in this way, but it is critical to your success in managing your pain.

Tension and numbness can also be caused by the thoughts that you have at the time you experience an emotion (e.g., frustration) or stressor (e.g., dealing with a particular person). When you experience stress, in addition to paying attention to your body, try to catch what you are thinking. Thoughts are fleeting, and it takes practice to catch them. But this skill, too, is critical to practice. We will return to the role of thoughts and feelings in pain management in lesson 7. For now it is important to simply understand that thoughts and feelings can increase muscular tension and pain and that awareness of bodily sensations and thoughts can help relax muscles and reduce pain.

Uncertainty and Fear

Fears of open spaces, anxiety while traveling in cars and other enclosed vehicles, fear of crossing bridges, and heightened tension in shopping malls are all quite common in the general population. These fears can be accompanied by dizziness, shortness of breath, and rapid heart beat. This in turn can lead to further anxiety and avoidance of situations that cause these distressing sensations. However, avoidance of travel, outings, and social situations can increase feelings of isolation and actually increase stress over the long run.

Other fears are less specific and can be experienced as "free floating" anxiety. Common concerns our patients have found to underlie these fears are (a) their pain will never end; (b) their pain or underlying condition will worsen; (c) they will become progressively more disabled and dependent on others; and (d) people won't believe how bad their pain really is.

Such fears and thoughts often occur spontaneously and are accompanied by rapid, shallow breathing. This type of breathing can occur without awareness and can also increase muscle tension directly and lead to anxiety or panic attacks. Later in this lesson, we will teach you some skills to help you breathe through these stress-provoking situations and feelings so as not to increase your stress and pain.

Loss of Concentration

Tension, as well as pain, often interfere with concentration and memory. Also, some medications for pain can have these effects. These may be dose dependent (i.e., the more medication taken, the worse the side effects), so lowering dosages can sometimes help with these cognitive problems. People with chronic pain often describe their state of mind as similar to walking around in a fog.

Have you felt a decrease in your ability to concentrate and remember things since your pain began? Do you feel sometimes as if your brain is in a fog? Has your pain affected your memory, your concentration, and your attention span?

Chronic Fatigue

Some people with chronic pain also feel a sense of "chronic fatigue" or constant tiredness. They start the day feeling tired, so they often wonder what's the sense in getting out of bed. Sitting or standing for a long period may feel daunting, and climbing the stairs seems like climbing a mountain. Every effort seems to be too much to bear. When they push themselves, they feel as if they are engaged in battle, with pressure in their chests and a racing heartbeat.

Much of this is the result of being physically unfit from restricting activity. Using fuel in appropriate ways makes the body more fuel-efficient. That is why the last lesson was so vitally important, even in terms of chronic fatigue.

Some people try to pep up their overloaded nervous system with stimulants (e.g., prescribed medication, nicotine, caffeine). This may help at the moment, but actually leads to more exhaustion later on.

This is because it is possible to artificially boost the exhausted body for a short time. Over time, however, these stimulants backfire, overwhelming the nervous system and creating more anxiety and stress. As people become physically dependent and require larger quantities of these stimulants to get the same effect, they become more exhausted still.

Sleep Problems

It seems strange to many of our patients that despite their fatigue, their sleep is not refreshing. Many have trouble falling asleep and staying asleep. Their sleep may be fitful, and they wake up more tired than they were when they went to bed. Some people are not even aware their sleep is disturbed until they ask their partner or room with someone else temporarily (e.g., on an outing or a retreat).

Think about yourself for a moment. How would you describe your pattern of sleep? Do you toss and turn a lot? Do you wake up feeling just as tired as when you went to sleep?

Digestive Problems

Some of our patients report problems with swallowing, feeling "too full," being constipated, having frequent diarrhea, losing their appetite, overeating, or alternating over- with under-eating. They often report an increase in weight, most often because of inactivity and extra snacking to fill up the space pleasurable activities used to occupy. This extra weight makes their bodies less fuel efficient and contributes to tension and fatigue. It also results in feelings of unattractiveness. For example, one of our male patients used to enjoy ballroom dancing, but he no longer went dancing because of the increased visible weight he carried. Many women turn down routine social invitations that could potentially increase their energy because they are embarrassed about their weight gain.

Changes in the Immune System

Additionally, our pain patients have reported increased problems with infection and allergies as well as a heightened susceptibility to colds and flu. This typically results from a combination of inactivity, poor diet, daily stress, and the stress of coping with chronic pain as opposed to the original cause of their pain.

Whereas the immune system must fight germs all of the time, the stressors and symptoms described in this section deplete the immune system's arsenal in such a way that the person who suffers from chronic pain may actually be more likely to incur other illnesses. Relaxation can help replenish this arsenal in addition to helping decrease pain directly. But how exactly does one learn how to relax?

Learning to Relax

We have already mentioned two major skills involved in learning to relax: bodily awareness of stress and emotions and mental awareness of thoughts that accompany stress. Whereas we will have much more to say about thoughts in later lessons, in this lesson we will focus on bodily relaxation.

You probably already "try" to relax. Some methods are better than others. Think of whether you use any of the following methods.

Alcohol and Other Drugs

Alcohol (yes, alcohol is a drug), antianxiety prescription drugs (e.g., valium, clonazepam), and some antidepressant drugs relax the muscles. The result is that feelings of arousal, worry, and tension may be temporarily reduced or suppressed. However, these muscle-relaxing drugs have the disadvantage of addiction or tolerance. (Tolerance means that you continually need more of the drugs to achieve the same effect.)

If you have been taking such drugs for more than a week, do not stop taking them (with the exception of alcohol, perhaps) unless you are under the supervision of a physician. You cannot stop most drugs rapidly or "cold turkey" without your body responding in alarming or harmful ways (e.g., seizures).

If you start to reduce these drugs even under the supervision of a physician, or even if you stop drinking alcohol abruptly, you may notice some unpleasant side effects (e.g., headache, sweating, flu-like symptoms, difficulty sleeping or concentrating). Even stopping caffeine can have strong effects. One of us (Dennis Turk), a frequent caffeine consumer, reduced his caffeine intake all at once and began feeling like he was in a fog. He was unable to concentrate and had a throbbing headache for 10 days.

So, it is better to gradually wean yourself (with the advice of your physician) from any prescription and nonprescription drugs you are using to reduce stress. (Note that we are not talking about specific pain medications here—these are a totally different topic.)

Television and Reading

Many people use television to tune out. People, in general, tend to unwind in front of the television at night. But more than an hour or so of television ceases to be relaxing and becomes a substitute for living.

Others become "hooked" on romance novels or mysteries. Again, these are healthy outlets if they are used moderately. Reading in bed for 3 hours on a regular basis, however, can be as unhealthy as watching television for the same length of time.

Computer Games and the Internet

Many people become "addicted" to playing computer games (both interactive and solitary), to Internet gambling, and to shopping online. Time seems to fly when they are online, and hours go by in a sort of haze. Not only does excessive involvement (i.e., over 1 hour a day) in these activities decrease social skills and increase inactivity, it also can cause repetitive stress injuries. Thus, they can add insult to injury for people already experiencing chronic pain.

Relaxation Exercises

Some of our patients had tried relaxation exercises before they consulted us, but these activities didn't seem to work. At times this was because they had chosen a form of relaxation that didn't fit their personality, and at others times it was because they didn't stay with the process long enough.

Some people benefit from relaxation involving imagery (mental pictures), others benefit from tapes (video or audio), and still others need some physical activity while they relax (e.g., floating in water, gentle stretching). If you choose a method that is not right for you, you will be unlikely to enjoy it or keep practicing long enough to achieve results.

Learning to relax takes practice. Patients with serious heart problems, for example, are asked to do daily relaxation exercises consistently for 90 days before they can expect to see results. This is because real relaxation seems deceptively simple, but it is really a hard skill to learn. You must learn what method is right for you and then you must practice, practice, and practice.

If you do practice consistently, you are likely to feel out of sorts when you miss a session, or feel like you do when you have forgotten to brush your teeth. In this lesson we will focus on a few of the many ways to learn to relax. If the ways we have described do not work for you, do not give up. There are a variety of audio relaxation tools and also classes in many communities that teach relaxation in different ways, including in groups. You may be the type of person that benefits from relaxation in a group!

There are many different ways to relax your body and your mind. We describe several different methods below. There is no one best way to relax. The important thing is to find some means of relaxing that is comfortable for you and to use these activities on a daily basis. They should become just as much a part of your daily routine as brushing your teeth.

Systematic Muscle Relaxation

As you learned earlier in this lesson, there are muscles that are under your control even if you are not aware of it at the moment. Skeletal muscles fall into this category. There are however, also muscles that do their work more automatically and without conscious awareness (e.g., the internal muscles of the digestive system [stomach and bowels] and your heart muscle, among others). With practice, however, you can gain some control over many of these muscles as well. We have provided some exercises to help you relax muscles in Appendix 3.1.

Breathing Correctly

Many people are "chest breathers." That is, they suck in their abdomens and expand their chests with each in breath. This may be particularly true for women because in Western culture they are taught early in life that the "proper" posture is one in which the abdomen is flat at all times.

This posture is difficult to maintain when you are truly relaxing. Diaphragmatic breathing, which produces the truly relaxing breath, requires the stomach to move in and out with each breath. If you want to observe natural diaphragmatic breathing, watch infants when they breathe. Their tummies move gently in and out with each breath.

Many people also become shallow, chest breathers because of prolonged anxiety, stress, and tension. When tensed, your breathing naturally becomes faster, more shallow, and from the chest. Stress tends to increase tension in the abdominal area, so the diaphragm cannot contract completely and the abdominal wall cannot move out when taking a breath. Only the chest expands as a result, causing further tension.

The first step in learning to truly relax, the one you must master before you proceed further, is to practice diaphragmatic breathing. Brief periods of diaphragmatic breathing provide for your body's energy needs in two ways. First, this type of breathing is best able to remove the carbon dioxide from your blood. At the same time, it produces oxygen, both great sources of energy. Second, breathing properly ensures beneficial massage of the abdominal organs. (This is why gentle yoga can be effective as well.)

Diaphragmatic breathing can bring about a feeling of calm and relaxation when it is properly practiced. To feel your diaphragm during breathing, place your hand just above your stomach, take a slow deep breath through your nose, and feel the movement of your hand as you do so. As you breathe out through your mouth slowly, you will find yourself relaxing without even trying. Longer and deeper breathing of this sort can make "normal" breathing easier and more relaxed

When first learning how to breathe in this way, it often helps to lie down on a cushioned floor, knees slightly bent, and to place your hands on your stomach. In this way, you can feel the abdomen rise when you breathe in and contract when you breathe out. Try practicing 10 minutes or so while you are doing something passive in the morning, afternoon, and evening, such as listening to the radio.

Exercise 3.1 that follows provides detailed instructions for practice.

Exercise 3.1. Controlled Breathing

Before you begin practicing, you may want to read over this exercise a few times. Some people find it helpful to tape record themselves reading the exercise and then play it back. You can try different methods. We recommend that you wear loose, comfortable clothing and that you find a quiet, relaxing place to practice.

First, lie on your back. Place your hands just above your navel or " belly button" Close your eyes and imagine a balloon inside your abdomen. Each time you breathe in, imagine the balloon filling with air. Each time you breathe out, imagine the balloon collapsing.

Now inhale slowly and deeply in through your nose. Let your abdomen rise as you breathe in to the count of 4 (slow, e.g., 4 seconds). Then, slowly (e.g., to the count of 4) exhale through your mouth, feeling your abdomen sink as you do so.

Try practicing 10 breaths about 3 to 4 times a day. Once you have been able to do this, on the next day, with each slow breath in, focus on a single word such as CALM; on the out breath think of a related word, such as RELAX. Some people who belong to a religion or spiritual practice, find two words from their faith to focus on. If none of these options appeal to you, simply repeat BREATHING IN on the in breath and BREATHING OUT on the out breath.

Try to stay with the words you have chosen, which may be more difficult than at first appears. When your mind wanders, gently bring it back to your word as you breath in and out. If you are still having difficulty, try to choose a short word or shorten the word you have chosen and focus on each letter. For example, if you have chosen the word *calm*, as you breath in you would focus on each letter:

C

A

L

M

Once you have mastered this, you can begin to focus specifically on relaxing the muscle group that is easiest for you to relax. The next day, add another muscle group. Gradually work up to 15 minutes of controlled breathing, focusing, and relaxation. As you get better and better at this, you can try it out even when you are not sitting or lying down but are more active. In fact, some people find this exercise easier when they are stretching or slowly walking. In this way, you can take brief, mini-relaxations for a few seconds or minutes at any time.

We have included visualization exercises at the end of this lesson (see Appendix 3.2). You can try these out and see how they work for you.

Remember, becoming more skilled at controlled, relaxed breathing may take some time. So, don't be discouraged if what initially sounds easy is, in fact, a bit difficult. Many of us have a running monologue or dialogue in our heads most of the time, and it takes practice to quiet this voice.

You also may not feel immediate results. The body is not used to this kind of practice. It barely remembers infancy, when this kind of breathing came naturally. With practice, your body will begin to trust your mind again, and some days you will find these exercises both effortless *and* rewarding.

Try each of the different techniques discussed in this lesson and find the ones that are most helpful to you. You may find that different methods work better for you at different times. One man we treated became so good at diaphragmatic breathing that he taught and coached his pregnant wife so that she could control her breathing during the delivery of their first child and thus experience less pain.

Attention Diversion

Another way of achieving true relaxation is through diversion. Those who suffer from chronic pain naturally tend to focus on their bodies, on how severe the pain is, and on how much they can or cannot do. This is human nature. We each have the untapped ability, however, to attend to other things, at least some of the time. You can consider some ways to use your intentional focus to distract yourself when your pain is difficult to bear.

Many of our patients reply when we say this, "I can't distract myself. My pain is too severe." Here, we gently suggest that they try out some of the exercises and see what happens. We remind them that controlling attention when you have pain is difficult, and it helps to admit when things are difficult. And, we tell them that they will not experience immediate relief. Effective distraction, like controlled breathing, takes time and practice.

There are several ways to relax by diverting attention. The way diversion works with pain is based on the principle that we cannot focus on everything that is going on around us all the time. For example, while you are reading this lesson some sounds are likely going on in the background. Stop for a moment and listen. What do you hear? It might be the sound of the fan on your air conditioner or heater. It might be the wind blowing outside your window, traffic noises outside your home, or the ticking of a clock.

In the same way, there are feelings within our body that we fail to pay attention to all of the time. For example, you may have a watch on your wrist or ring on your finger. If you do, focus on how they feel against your skin. How about your socks or shoes? How do they feel? How does your back feel against the chair, couch, or bed on which you are reading. You may not notice these sensations until they are the focus of your attention

The important thing about this is to realize that all of these sensations are always going on, but out of habit we do not pay attention to them. This is because attention can be likened to watching a television or listening to the radio. All of the stations are there all of the time, but we can only tune into one station at a time.

When it comes to our pain, many people do not realize the power of focus and attention, particularly distraction. By distraction, we can choose what will be the focus of our attention for a specific period of time.

You have probably made use of attention diversion or distraction without even realizing it. You might read books or magazines, study religious materials, listen to music, work on a hobby, or listen to someone when they call to talk on the telephone. Sometimes when you do these activities you may even lose track of the time or where you are. In each of these cases, your attention is highly focused and you are likely not aware of many things going on around you.

We do not suggest that you should try distracting yourself all of the time, but there are times when distraction can help you feel a greater sense of control, create relaxation, and reduce the intensity of your pain. It is important to remember that you have at least some control over the focus of your attention. It is fine to be skeptical that you will be able to distract yourself. However, it is worth your effort to try.

Spiritual Focus: Meditation and Prayer

One way to divert attention from pain and induce a state of relaxation is to focus on some spiritual word, phrase, or prayer. When we discussed controlled breathing earlier, we mentioned that spiritual words can be used in conjunction with this type of breathing to help you relax. Prayer by itself or a focus on a religious figure such as Jesus, Mohammed, Buddha, or the spiritual being some call a *higher power* can be tremendously calming. Others find focusing on a sense of oneness with nature to be helpful. If this kind of focus appeals to you, you can focus on whatever you find most meaningful and relaxing.

Sensory Focus

We also tell our patients that if their pain, worries, or seemingly insoluble problems have kept them upset for a long time, it is not possible to let these difficulties go all at once. We ask them to practice visualizing one pleasant experience for a period of time. They are instructed to reach into their memories and recall a happy or peaceful time. They close their eyes and focus on each visual aspect of that scene. Then we ask them to focus on the sounds and smells associated with that scene, as well as the tactile memories—what the sun felt like if it was a summer scene, what the cold felt like, if it was winter. Try this now, at least once, for a few minutes.

It can also be helpful to see yourself in pleasant places to which you may never have gone:

◆ Picture yourself in the cool of dusk, sitting at the edge of a lake. Look at how the water reflects the light from the moon, feel the cool breeze against your skin, and hear the birds off in the distance.
◆ Picture yourself walking through a park on a beautiful autumn day. Hear the breeze rustling through the tall trees. Feel your feet sinking into the soft ground as the golden red, yellow, and orange leaves rustle beneath you.
◆ Picture yourself lying on an uncrowded beach at the ocean. Feel the sun on your face. Hear the breaking of the waves. See the horizon line as you look in the distance. Enjoy the feeling of space around you. Sit up and watch the different tints of blue, green, and gray in the sea. Enjoy the clear blue sky. Perhaps have a cold drink or Popsicle. Taste it. Savor each drop. Which drink or flavor did you choose?

We are sure that you can think of many other scenes once you get the idea. Such relaxing images have a direct effect on muscle tension. Focusing on these can take your mind off your pain, even for only a moment.

The particular image that you use in coping with pain is *not* the most important thing. The most important thing is to be *involved* in the image, so that all of your attention is focused on the image and the sensations. Whenever possible, make use of all of your senses—vision, hearing, touch, taste, and smell.

As in the breathing exercises, your attention may wander from time to time, and you may occasionally find yourself dwelling on unpleasant sensations. But you can gently bring your attention back to the pleasant image or scene when you notice that your attention has wandered.

As you first start this practice or when you practice on bad days, you may still be somewhat aware of the discomfort or pain. But these will gradually fade into the background as you focus on the sensations associated with the scene. The pain may not disappear, but it may be more like the ticking of a clock or the sound of a fan—noticeable but not too irritating.

What would be a pleasant scene for you? What would you include? Pleasant images bring with them a feeling of safety. (In Appendix 3.2 at the end of this lesson, we have included a detailed sample of a scene that many people find pleasant.) You might read this over and then try to experience it yourself. Once again, you may wish to make a tape of yourself reading this scene. Perhaps someone you are very comfortable with may be willing to read the scene and record it for you.

If you have trouble coming up with a scene, look at pictures in nature, island travel, or pictoral magazines. Many libraries have such magazines available. Even if you don't use the scene in a focused exercise, just looking at such pictures can be relaxing. The same is true with watching nature channels on television.

Keep in mind when you use such scenes that there is no reason for you to feel *locked in* to any one image. If you find the scene that you are using to be ineffective or even distressing, you can easily switch to another scene. Some images may inadvertently unconsciously recall distressful times in your life that you may have forgotten. Also, some images fade and become less vivid after a while.

You can elaborate on such images by including other senses, such as the tastes and smells associated with a picnic in a lake or forest scene. You might also bring movement into the picture. For example, picture yourself dancing alone on the beach. There is no limit to what you can include, as long as the image is not distressing.

At times you may find that you can maintain one very detailed image for a long time. At other times, your mind may flit from one image to another or you may find images merging and blending. This is fine, as long as you are relaxed. There is no right way or wrong way to do this. Try to find what works best for you.

Creating a Pleasant and Safe Home Environment

In addition to creating peaceful spaces in your body, it is important to create a peaceful refuge in your home. Do you have a favorite room or a part of a room where you feel most peaceful? Are you able to set limits on family members so that you have time alone in your "space"? Think about this and how to approach family members (if needed) to safeguard your haven for at least part of the day. Even an hour can do wonders.

Here are some experiences that our patients have reported as being refreshing and refueling as they manage their pain.

◆ I nestle myself in my most comfortable chair and put on my favorite music. Sometimes I choose music that suits my mood. If I feel sad, I allow myself to listen to melancholy music. If I feel peppy, I play something lively. I really try to listen to the music. In particular, I resist the urge to do something else at the same time I am listening.

◆ In the evening, I take a warm bath or shower at around 8:00 p.m. Then I put on my favorite pajamas. I choose relaxing reading material. Books of meditations (e.g., daily readings) and children's books are my favorites. Then I settle into a comfortable chair with good lighting and light a candle with a lavender scent. After reading for about a half hour, I am ready to go to sleep.

◆ I find poetry to be a great way to relax. I try to read passages in the rhythm the author intended. Sometimes I listen to poems on cassette tapes or CDs.

Besides alone time, many people find the company of good friends in their relaxing space to be a great solace. As several of our patients told us,

◆ I always seek the company of people with whom I can be my real self. I invite them over in the evening in winter, light a fire, put on soft music, and fix a pot of decaffeinated tea. With some friends, I may offer a glass of wine. Then I try to simply be present with them in the moment. If I find myself talking too much, I try to remember that listening is more relaxing than talking at these times.

◆ It took a while, but I finally convinced my husband to spend 15 minutes just relaxing on the couch with me. No television. Sometimes we listen to old radio programs that have been recorded—nothing stressful (like the news of today). Sometimes we just listen to music that we both enjoy. Now, my husband looks forward to our relaxing time as much as I do.

◆ I asked my wife to spend time with me in the evening. Just nestling together. No sexual demands, just tender touch and caressing. She was leery at first. But now she understands that I just want to hold her and be held. I'm not trying to set up a prelude to sex. Interestingly, though, our sex life at other times has improved as a result.

The theme of all these patients' experience is that relaxing means not "doing" or "having" but simply "being." They also illustrate the importance of letting go of expectations and approaching each period of relaxation with an open mind and an open heart. There are no rights and wrongs, no shoulds or musts, no measures by which they rate their period of relaxation or its results. These patients have learned that despite pain they can learn to enjoy the moment, without having to achieve anything.

Really Enjoying Food

Sometimes when we are in pain, we have no appetite. It is hard to even think about eating, let alone enjoying a nutritious meal. At other times, we may use food as an anesthetic. We eat mindlessly to take our minds off our pain. Really planning a nutritious meal and eating in a slow relaxed way may seem foreign to us at those times. However, nutritious meals served in your nicest dishes, even if you are dining alone, can create a sense of peace and relaxation, as well as contributing to good health.

Maybe you use food in unhealthy ways. If you do, perhaps just once a week you can make one meal something special. Plan the menu, and set aside time to set the table so as to create a "dining atmosphere" (e.g., you can use candles, flowers, or your favorite dishes, placements, or table cloth). After you have prepared the meal, sit down and really take time to savor each bite of food. Some people find it relaxing to have some soft music in the background. Reading while eating, however, tends to distract one from the pleasure of eating. If this seems too much for you right now, try doing the same with a snack of fresh fruit in the middle of the day this week.

Enjoying a relaxed meal or snack not only induces relaxation, it also aids digestion. After the meal or snack is over, take time to have decaffeinated coffee or tea. If you are alone, perhaps you can use this time to think about next week's special meal or tomorrow's snack. Even planning the meal or snack can be relaxing and can be a helpful distraction from pain.

Try this for a few weeks. If you find that it relaxes you, you can increase the number of meals in which you truly enjoy your food in the weeks to come.

Enjoying Nature and Other People

Pain often gives one a feeling of being imprisoned, isolated, and alone. To decrease the feeling of being a "shut in," try to plan an outing that is not too taxing and that involves being in a natural environment. Maybe there is a park or some woods in your area, or maybe you are fortunate enough to be near a river, lake, or even the ocean. If it is winter, dress in layers, so you can adjust to the temperature as needed. Perhaps you will only stay 5 minutes at first. Eventually you may find yourself staying longer.

If it is too cold or hot, perhaps you can people-watch at a mall, coffee shop, or bookstore. Some people like just to be around people without having to necessarily interact with them.

Give yourself options. Try to get out of the house at least once a day at first, even if only for a few minutes. Try this for at least a week. Then, you can adjust the frequency and length of outings to fit your particular situation.

Giving Yourself Room to Breathe

What we have described so far is only part of the large number of relaxing activities. Others include massage, fishing, sitting in the sun (with sunscreen), or going to an outdoor café for a glass of iced tea in the summer. (We have listed more activities on pp. 89–90 at the end of lesson 4.)

None of these activities needs to cost much money. The most you need is gas for the car or some change to buy a cup of coffee, tea, or a bottled water. And you'll need one other thing: patience.

It's odd to think that you have to be patient to learn to "be" and to do the simplest things. But it is true. Give yourself the gift of relaxation, even if it takes a while to find what relaxes you most. The nonactivity you choose is not as important as giving yourself permission to experiment, to forget your worries, and to find room to breathe and get to know yourself again.

Summary

You can create your own ways of relaxing, just by practice. If you are better able to relax, despite the pain, you will have increased energy, a longer attention span, and a greater ability to concentrate. Over the course of a day, alternating what you have learned in this lesson (relaxation) with what you have learned in the previous lesson (increased activities) can improve your life immeasurably.

When you are in chronic pain, you may feel these lessons are too simple or too basic to help. You may wonder how they will help you decrease your pain. With this in mind, let's recap some of the main benefits of learning to relax:

◆ If your muscles are tense, you use energy that can be better spent on the things you want to do or enjoy.
◆ If your muscles are relaxed, you produce energy—physical, mental, and emotional.
◆ When you balance activity with relaxation, you learn to hear more clearly what your body is saying to you. Therefore, you will not do more than you are able to, but you will not do less.
◆ With the peace that comes from maintaining a proper energy balance, you become able to let go of things that are truly not in your control.

Coping with pain requires a lot of energy—mental, physical, and emotional. When activity is balanced with relaxation, you put money in your energy bank. When this equation gets out of balance, you withdraw money from the bank. Pretty soon, your account is overdrawn and your pain levels increase. As a result, you can become oversensitive to stimuli and experience chronic fatigue and sleep problems.

When your energy account is flush, you will find that the pain or your experience of it will be less. Your immune system will be strengthened, and you will experience less fear and better concentration.

Activities That Can Help

Critical Activities

1. Controlled breathing exercise. Practice controlled breathing at least twice a day every day this week. Start with 2 minutes the first day, then add a minute each day thereafter. Record your experiences in your journal or notebook.

Some people find it helpful to have a written script that they can follow as they learn to practice controlled breathing. The following is one suggested script:

◆ Sit or lie down in a comfortable, relaxed position.
◆ Inhale slowly and deeply through your nose.
◆ Hold your breath and count up to 4 at 1-second intervals ("a thousand 1", "a thousand 2", "a thousand 3", "a thousand 4") and then slowly exhale through your mouth.
◆ As you hold your breath, think of a single word such as "C–A–L–M" or P–E–A–C–E," to help free your mind from distracting or stressful thoughts. You can also say "breathe in" as you're breathing in and "breathe out" as you're breathing out.
◆ As you exhale, let your chest and stomach muscles relax, and if seated drop your shoulders.

Repeat this cycle at least three times for approximately 3 to 5 minutes.

2. Identifying pleasant scenes. In your journal or notebook, describe a scene or situation that you have found pleasant (e.g., a walk in a meadow). Try to include as much detail as you can—where you are, what you see, what you hear, what you smell, what you taste, and who is with you (if anyone). Once you have prepared this example, try to focus on the details as you do the controlled breathing exercises described earlier. Relax by slowly inhaling and exhaling and focusing on one of the pleasant scenes you have written down.

3. Choose a day in the week to plan for your special meal or snack. Allow enough time for rest after preparation of the meal so that you will truly enjoy it.

Optional Activities

4. Thinking back in time, recent or long ago, answer the following questions:

◆ Where and with whom have you been able to relax? Did you relax more alone or with others?

◆ Were there certain activities (or nonactivities) that made you more relaxed?
◆ Were there certain thoughts, worries, or people who interrupted your relaxation? In the same vein, were there thoughts or people who made you feel more relaxed?
◆ Were there particular times of the day when you were best able to relax? Morning, afternoon, evening?

5. Some people have more difficulty than others with relaxation. If you do, you might consider the following:

◆ Forgetting to relax: The use of charts to record activities (described earlier) and keeping these in a visible place can help.
◆ Mind wandering to worrisome thoughts: Redirect your thoughts by focusing on something pleasant.
◆ Falling asleep: This is not a bad thing. If it happens frequently, try to find another time of day to relax.
◆ Difficulty concentrating on breathing and guided relaxation: Make an audiotape or have someone make one for you. You can then play the tape and concentrate on the voice and the instructions on the tape.

6. Make a daily schedule in which you experiment with a good balance between exertion, diversion, and relaxation. As with other exercises, you may find it helpful to create or record your progress:

	Monday	Tuesday	Wednesday	Thursday	Friday	Saturday
Morning	____ min	____ min	____ min	____ min	____ min	____ min
Afternoon	____ min	____ min	____ min	____ min	____ min	____ min
Evening	____ min	____ min	____ min	____ min	____ min	____ min
Total	____ min	____ min	____ min	____ min	____ min	____ min

Appendix 3.1
Progressive Muscle Relaxation

Some people find it helpful to have a script for focusing while relaxing:

Now, close your eyes for a few moments and focus on how your body feels. Move your focus to different parts of your body and see if you can notice any tension in any particular part. How about where you have the most pain? Can you detect any tension there? You may feel more pain when you focus on it. That's natural. You may not feel any tension at first. That is natural as well. Just let what is "be" without judging the exercise or yourself.

If you notice tension in any part of your body, compare that sensation to body parts that don't feel so tense. Now just let the tension go, let it drift away. It might be helpful to imagine the tense body part feeling more and more like the parts of your body that do not feel tense. Now, curl the toes of your left foot toward the bottom of your foot or the floor.

◆ Hold this tense position. Feel the tightness in your ankle and the sole of your foot. As you feel it, note how it feels exactly.
◆ Now, relax your foot by moving your toes away from the bottom of your foot or the floor.
◆ Let your toes relax. Let the tension drain from your toes. Feel the warm comfortable sensations of relaxation that you have been able to produce.
◆ Pay attention to these sensations and notice how they differ from the cramped or tight sensations of tensing your muscles.
◆ Repeat with right foot, but replace the first sentence with, "Pull the toes of your left foot up toward your face."

Continue using these instructions, replacing the first sentence with the instructions below, and alternating right to left where applicable:

Now, tense the muscles in your left thigh by pressing hard against your other leg. Relax your left thigh . . . (Right)

◆ Tighten the muscles of your buttocks by pulling them toward each other. Relax your buttocks.
◆ Tighten the muscles of your stomach as if you were trying to protect yourself from being punched. Relax your stomach muscles.
◆ Pull your shoulder blades toward each other. Relax your shoulder blades.
◆ Hunch your shoulders toward your ears. Relax your shoulders.
◆ Press the upper part of your right arm against your right side. Relax the upper right arm muscles . . . Do the same with the left arm.

- Make a tight fist with your right hand. Relax your right hand . . . Do the same with the left hand.
- Push the back of your head hard against the floor or chair to tighten your neck muscles. Relax your neck muscles.
- Clench your teeth together, push your tongue against the roof of your mouth, and smile to expose as many teeth as you can. Relax your mouth.
- Squint your eyes tightly shut, and wrinkle your nose. Relax your face.
- Raise your eyebrows as high as you can to wrinkle your forehead. Relax your face.

If you notice any tension left in a particular part of the body, compare those sensations to parts of the body that feel relaxed. Let the tense body part drift into the same feeling as the relaxed body part.

Appendix 3.2
Example of a Pleasant Image

Read this example through and then try to imagine yourself in this or a similar scene. It may be helpful to audiotape yourself reading or have someone you care about make a tape for you.

Picture yourself standing by the shore of a large lake, looking out across an expanse of blue water and beyond, to the far shore. Immediately in front of you stretches a small beach and behind you a grassy meadow. The sun is shining brightly and feels very pleasant, bathing the landscape in a shimmering brightness.

It is a gorgeous spring day. The sky is pale blue, with a few soft, fluffy clouds gently drifting by. The breeze is blowing gently, just enough to make the trees sway and to make ripples in the grass. Feel the wind on your cheeks. You have this perfect day entirely to yourself, with nothing to do and nowhere to go.

You have a blanket, a towel, and a bottle of lemonade with you, and you carry them lightly as you walk through the meadow. You find a spot, spread the blanket, and set your lemonade aside.

Now, lie down on your blanket. It is a soft spot, and you feel comfortable. There are only a few gentle noises: a bird chirping, the breeze occasionally blowing over the meadow. The quiet is very peaceful and relaxing. Tell yourself to just relax and take it easy. Think about the warm, beautiful day.

Feel the sun on your body. Totally let go of your cares and enjoy the sensations you are feeling now.

After a while, you hear the water lapping at the shore in the distance. You take a drink of your lemonade, savoring the sour sweetness.

You walk toward it, feeling the soft, lush grass of the meadow under your feet. You reach the sand of the beach and feel the different texture under your feet.

The sand is warm but not too warm. Let any tension remaining drain into the sand.

Now visualize yourself walking into the water slowly. Feel the refreshing wetness as the water reaches your ankles. As you feel ready, walk in the water until it is up to your knees. The sun has warmed the water pleasantly. It is almost like being in a bath.

As the breeze continues to blow gently, you look around. You have this lovely spot all to yourself.

Far across the lake you can see a sailboat, tiny in the distance. It is so far away that you can just make out the white sail jutting up from the blue water. You stay in the water as long as you like.

When you are ready, return to your spot at the meadow. Take another drink of lemonade. Lie down and just enjoy.

It is a warm spring day, and the sun has grown hotter, but it is still pleasant—it is a comfortable, dry heat. Your body absorbs this heat and further relaxes.

As the day progresses, you are partly in the sun and partly in the shade. Feel the difference on your body. Look up at the sky and watch the clouds. Sometimes they seem to form animals or things.

You can hear the sound of a bird gently singing in a tree nearby. You smell the sweet grass around you. You are totally relaxed.

If you'd like, take more time to continue imagining pleasant scenes and sensations, enjoying the positive feelings you have been able to bring forth.

Are You Always Tired? Ways to Combat Fatigue

In your hierarchy of values, nothing can have higher priority than health,
And if you find time for watching television but not for walking, swimming or jogging,
You are violating the most important rule of time management,
which is to do the most important things first.
—Edward C. Bliss

Chronic pain is usually accompanied by chronic fatigue. Many of our patients report that they do not get a good night's sleep, and that they doze off and on during the day. As a result, they lack energy, feel weak, and experience tiredness, even after mild exertion. So, it is not only the pain that causes you to limit your activities, it may also be an enduring sense of fatigue and weakness.

This kind of tiredness can be every bit as disabling as the pain itself. You may drag yourself through the day. You feel as if you can't even face minor chores. Everything seems like too much. Without really meaning to, you tell everyone by your behavior, "Leave me alone."

The troubling thing is that this sense of fatigue never seems to go away, even when you are inactive and do little or nothing. Even though you believe you hear your body saying "take it easy, sit down, or lie down for an hour," you're not sure that that's the right thing to do. You wonder if you can trust your body at all.

In this lesson you will learn the following:

◆ What causes extreme fatigue and how it can be overcome.
◆ How your sleep, eating, and activity patterns affect your store of energy.
◆ How certain lifestyle habits rob you of energy.
◆ What is most important in restoring your energy balance so that you can feel rested again.

Your Body's Energy System

Your own energy system can be likened to a power generator or a battery. A generator needs fuel to create power. If there is no fuel, even the strongest generator is unable to produce power. The fuel for your body is created in tiny energy centers in your cells (*mitochondria*). These mitochondria need a small amount of energy to be able to function adequately. Like a car battery, your own "battery" can only be charged when you still have some energy in reserve.

When you are too tired, your body does not even have enough energy to produce the minimal charge you need to be active. It is important, therefore, to maintain sufficient energy reserves. If you go to sleep exhausted, there will be no electrical charge to allow your battery or energy centers to operate. That is why you may wake up tired even before you begin your day.

Let's begin with a simple suggestion. As we noted in earlier lessons, it is important that you learn to know and respect your own limits. In lesson 2, you learned to pace your activities so you can conserve your energy. A good balance of activity and rest throughout the day will ensure that there is still fuel left in reserve for your power generator to operate throughout the night. If you skipped over or skimmed lesson 2, this might be a good time to read or review it.

There are many kinds of tiredness. The following sections describes three kinds: emotional, physical, and nutritional.

Emotional Tiredness

After strenuous physical activity it is normal to feel some fatigue. If you have worked on the suggested activities so far, you are well acquainted with this normal sense of physical tiredness. There is, however, another sort of fatigue that is often ignored—emotional tiredness. This kind of tiredness occurs when you have to do boring, uninteresting, or repetitive work. It can also occur when you are alone and isolated or when you are annoyed and frustrated. It most often occurs in relation to other people. For example, as we will discuss in a later lesson, miscommunication and conflict with friends and family can create enormous emotional stress. This stress leads to emotional tiredness.

Being around someone who is tiring (e.g., complains, "yes, buts," always sees the glass is half empty, or talks nonstop) is not as rewarding as sitting quietly with a friend whom you value. Reading romance novels is not as satisfying as reading about inspiring figures.

Lack of success at what we try is an often unrecognized cause of emotional tiredness. It is exhausting and draining to continually feel as if one has failed or fallen short of expectations. This emotional tiredness often occurs with our chronic pain patients. When they begin becoming active and balancing rest with activity, they feel what they are doing does not amount to much. We remind them that there is a big difference between what they want to do eventually and what they are able to do in the present moment. Change evolves gradually, if it is to last.

Do you get annoyed with yourself and your progress? Do you feel frustrated? Do you get angry with yourself when you cannot do what you want to do? Many of our patients do. We explain to them that this constant annoyance and scolding of oneself increases feelings of fatigue.

For many, these feelings and fatigue are too quickly linked to the "amount" of activity. This is not always true. Quality of activity may be more important than quantity. For example, gamblers are able to stand for hours behind a coin-operated slot machine, without being bored or fatigued. Many have to virtually wrestle themselves away from the machine or go broke before they stop this repetitive action. (A similar activity with a strictly predictable result would be deadly boring and thus tiring.) Some of today's students (or adults) can spend hours in concentrated thought when they are playing computer games. When faced with necessary chores they do not like, they can become fatigued after a relatively brief period.

So, when considering progress, the quality, not the quantity, of activity needs to be taken into consideration. Playing solitaire at the computer for 2 hours is not as qualitatively good for a person as walking for 10 or even 5 minutes. Sitting in front of the television for 2 hours is not as qualitatively successful as doing a relaxation exercise for 5 or 10 minutes.

One way to avoid this kind of emotional fatigue is to define success on your own terms. When you are resting, choose to do things that really increase your self-worth or induce relaxation. When you are active, choose activities you look forward to doing, or people that you look forward to seeing. This is particularly important at the beginning of your efforts. Later, you can take on activities that may not initially engage you and give them a try.

Many people do not realize that these emotional factors can drain their energy and make them feel tired. You might have thought: "I do not understand why I am so tired, I have done practically nothing." With chronic pain, emotional fatigue invariably plays a role in chronic tiredness.

Physical Tiredness

As we noted in lesson 2, chronic pain affects your posture and especially the way in which and the extent to which you move about. You may have noticed that since your pain began you have moved more and more slowly and perhaps your posture has changed.

As we discussed in lesson 2, these changes occur because your muscle strength starts to weaken when you are inactive and your posture changes when you are trying to protect yourself from pain. These changes often lead to additional inactivity, weakness, and reduced

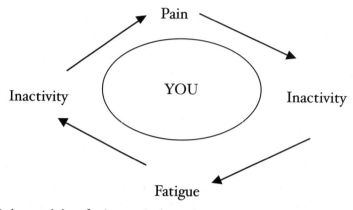

Figure 4.1. Pain–activity–fatigue circle.

strength. Thus, the vicious circle—pain causes inactivity and postural change; these lead to more pain; more pain leads to fatigue; and fatigue leads to inactivity, and so on (see Figure 4.1).

You may have found that increasing your activity level as we suggested in lesson 2 has increased your feelings of fatigue. In the short-term, this may be true. If you have been inactive for some time, your muscles are weak. However, if you gradually build up the amount of activity you perform, you will find that the increased muscle tone will allow you to do more for longer periods of time without a sense of exhaustion. (If you have done too much after reading lesson 2, you may feel more tired as well. Review your charts to see if you may have started at too high a level. Or, perhaps you did not allow enough rest between periods of activity.)

Please do not be disheartened if things are going slowly in terms of progress. This is to be expected. But if you stick with your plan, even if you have had to modify it, you will begin to notice improvements in your muscle flexibility, strength, and endurance that will allow you to do more with less pain and fatigue. The improvements will occur at different rates for different people.

A benefit of becoming active and exercising is that it helps the body increase the production of internal pain-relieving chemicals. Research has demonstrated that the body actually produces its own analgesics or pain reducers that are similar to morphine and are referred to as "*endorphins.*" Thus, endorphins are the body's natural pain reducers. This explains how as you increase your activities not only will you build up your muscular stamina but you may also experience a reduction in pain.

Many of our patients have suffered from chronic pain for a long time. It takes time to undo the effects of inactivity and to allow the body to increase its production of these natural pain reducers. As we tell our patients, be realistic. Do not expect change to occur over a few days or weeks. Stay with us for the long haul.

Nutritional Tiredness

Pain, discomfort, and resulting negative moods can have different effects on people. For some of our patients, appetite disappears. For others, appetite increases. Both eating too much and eating too little have a negative influence on energy levels.

How is your appetite? Do you eat three regular meals each day or six mini-meals? What about too frequent snacking of the nonnutritional kind? Have you lost or gained weight since your pain began?

If you eat too little, it may be because food has lost its appeal over time. Or you may not feel that you have the energy to prepare a meal. Perhaps your pain is so severe you feel you just can't make the effort. Or, perhaps you nibble snack foods throughout the day that do not require much preparation but have little nutritional value. Even here, you may feel you have to force yourself to eat.

When you do not eat enough of the right kinds of food, you receive too little of the right kind of fuel—fuel that can turn into consistent reserves of energy. Another disadvantage of eating too little or eating the wrong foods is that the muscle tissue breaks down. Less muscle means less power, and also less energy.

On the other hand, many of our patients report that their appetites have increased since their pain started. When we ask them what they are eating, we learn that it is usually their "comfort foods." They want comfort because of the pain, but also because they are often alone and bored. This is natural but dangerous.

For these eaters, between meal snacks are often a particular problem. The extra calories of snacks (usually something sweet or salty or buttery), cause them to gain weight. If they are inactive, this weight gain often skyrockets, because inactivity reduces the number of calories burned. For these inactive patients, even eating the same amount of food they ate before their chronic pain began can lead to increased weight. And, again, another vicious circle is created: pain leads to comfort eating; this leads to increased weight; increased weight leads to increased fatigue and inactivity; comfort eating begins again, and so on.

What can help? Because during the day you need energy, you need to begin eating three nutritious meals (or six mini-meals) regularly. Eat as little as possible between these meals or mini-meals. If you do require some snacks, consume fruit or raw vegetables with fat free dip instead of cookies or potato chips.

Another problem all of us face is that we are often on automatic pilot when it comes to eating. As described in lesson 3, many times we eat without even being aware that we are eating. We taste the first bite, but we space out or do other things while eating so we really don't taste much of the rest. Try eating more mindfully and slowly. Try to savor every bite. You may find that you are full on much less food this way.

If you are a comfort food eater, before turning to food, ask yourself, What am I feeling? Consider the following emotions: anger, irritation, or frustration; sadness, disappointment or depression; grief; hopelessness, helplessness; hurt or fear; worry or anxiety; passivity or boredom. Just recognizing which emotion you might be feeling at the moment you feel like having a donut can help you make different choices.

If you still feel like snacking, ask yourself, *"Does this snack contain good calories?" Will it provide me with an immediate "lift" only to let me down later? Will it provide me with energy or will it simply add to my weight?" Are there any substitutes that might do the trick (e.g., sugar free cocoa and whole wheat toast instead of a chocolate bar)?*

Finally, if you are having trouble with weight, consider eating your main meal (or mini meals) during the middle of the day. At night, we don't require as many calories, so a light evening meal and a small nutritious "bedtime snack" (e.g., a bowl of oatmeal or a cup of skim milk) may be all that you need.

Tips for Losing Weight

Our patients have shared with us a number of tips for losing weight and thus gaining energy:

◆ Eat a balanced diet.
◆ Use nutritional counts (e.g., such as calories, fats, carbohydrates, or protein).
◆ Avoid "crash diets" or "fad diets."
◆ Lose weight slowly so that you can learn how to eat to maintain your weight later.
◆ Decrease size of portions and use a small plate. (It's amazing the difference a small plate makes!)
◆ Exercise before you eat.
◆ Eat slowly; savor each bite. Find a nutrition "buddy," "partner," or weight loss support group (some are free).
◆ Eat more fruits and vegetables.

Dietary and Nutritional Supplements

We are frequently asked about the benefits of vitamins and dietary supplements for fatigue and chronic pain. Although many people report on the benefits of these supplements, we know of no consistent scientific evidence to support these claims at the current time. This does not mean that some supplements are not useful; there is just not sufficient information to draw any firm conclusions yet.

One problem is that dietary supplements are not regulated, so it is nearly impossible to know what and what amount of any supplement is helpful. For example, omega 3 oil has been helpful for heart patients, but the amount of omega 3 in proportion to omega 6 oils in supplements varies widely among brands of this supplement. In addition, there is limited information about the interaction of the active ingredients contained in supplements and prescribed pain medications and over-the-counter drugs.

Claims for excessive benefits often appear in newspapers, magazines, television, and the Internet. Many people believe that if they are publicly endorsed, then they have been approved by some governmental or watchdog agency. This is not true. The U.S. government (Food and Drug Administration), for example, monitors claims for prescribed medication, but it does not oversee food supplements. Moreover, no agency controls what information appears on the Internet.

In short, be cautious of excessive claims for the benefits of dietary supplements, as these are often based on little scientific evidence. These claims often rely on personal testimonials that are used to help the company make a tidy profit. Endorsement by famous people (for example, a television or movie star, a retired athlete, or a doctor who stands to profit) does not mean the product will be helpful. If you have a personal physician who is knowledgeable about supplements, that is the person to ask.

Other Ways of Improving Sleep

A puzzling thing for many is that tiredness as a result of pain and fatigue does not automatically lead to deep and refreshing sleep. You may have noticed this yourself.

How would you describe your sleep? Consider the following questions: Is your sleep restless? Does your body more or less remain in a state of alarm throughout the night? Do you have problems falling asleep at night? Staying asleep? Do you have bad dreams or nightmares? Does your pain wake you up during the night? If your answer to one or more of these questions is yes, you almost surely do not feel rested when you wake up.

How is your general mood during the day? Consider the following questions: Are you often irritable? Do you feel sad for no apparent reason? Do you often feel like "giving up"? Have you lost interest in activities that you can still do? Do you sometimes feel "worthless"? Many people who suffer from chronic illness or experience chronic pain become depressed. This is not surprising. Who would not become depressed if, in addition to the "daily routine of life," they had to struggle with illness or pain every day? Who wouldn't be depressed if every day they were aware of the things that they were no longer able to do?

Lack of sleep and poor sleep quality can be a symptom of depression. It can also worsen the other symptoms of depression described above. So it is no surprise that when people do not get restful sleep, they often try prescribed or over-the-counter sleeping pills. Others turn to alcohol as a way of getting to sleep or staying asleep and avoiding feeling depressed. Unfortunately, these remedies, if used for more than 2 weeks, can actually worsen the sleep problem. Many of these drugs (yes, as noted, alcohol is a drug) are addictive if used daily over even a very short period of time. And they do not really solve the sleep problem; they only temporarily mask the symptoms.

Changing thoughts and behaviors can improve some symptoms of depression, and in a later lesson we will help you with that. But for now, let's continue with our discussion of sleep.

It is important to know that the amount of sleep you get and the quality of that sleep are not the same. This is because there are four stages of sleep, each with very different characteristics. In general, there is a light stage of sleep and a very deep sleep, in which dreaming often occurs. It is this deep sleep that is truly refreshing.

Sleep medication or alcohol may lead to light sleep throughout the night, so that when you awaken you notice that a number of hours have passed but you may still feel tired. And, again, there is the problem of dependence. If you feel desperate about your sleep right now, consult a physician who is trained to treat sleep problems (not all physicians are). If you can hold off for a while in terms of your sleep, the program described in this book, followed consistently and resolutely, should lead to a gradual but steady improvement in sleep patterns. In Exhibit 4.1 we have listed a number of things you can do to achieve the deepest levels of sleep. Some of these may be familiar to you already.

Although doing or not doing things on this list will help, be aware that just as you cannot "force" relaxation, you cannot "force" sleep. The only thing you can do is to consistently take our suggestions to heart (and do them!) over a period of time.

Our patients have also found the following suggestions to be helpful.

◆ *Cut back on your caffeine during the day.* Caffeine, as most people know, is a stimulant. That is why so many people "need" a cup of coffee to get them going in the morning (they also "need" it because their bodies become physically dependent on caffeine). Even people who know that caffeine "arouses" them, may not know that caffeine, even if consumed early in the day, can interfere with sleep. We don't suggest to our patients that they go off caffeine "cold turkey." First, keep a log of how many drinks that you have each day. Gradually cut back (e.g., cut out one caffeinated beverage one day; cut out that one and a second the next, and so on).

◆ *Design your own personalized bedtime ritual.* The human body likes a fixed rhythm and regularity. Sleep rituals involve consistently following the same steps before you go to bed. For example, some of our patients lay out their sleep clothes, read a meditation or other comforting short passage, and take a warm bath before they go

Exhibit 4.1. Do's and Don'ts for a Good Night's Sleep

Do's	Don'ts
Keep a neat and comfortable bedroom; change linens at least once a week; buy good pillows if you can afford them; choose a firm (not too hard or soft) mattress that does not squeak.	Have radios, TV's, stereos on in the bedroom; read in bed.
Relax before you go to bed; read in the living room; listen to soothing music.	Drink or eat caffeinated beverages or foods (e.g., coffee, tea, chocolate) after 2:00 p.m.
Keep your room at a temperature that helps with your sleep (depending on your age and gender, this may differ).	Drink alcohol after 7:00 p.m.
Have a set time to wake and go to sleep.	Take unscheduled naps during the day.
Reserve the bedroom for sleep or sexual activity.	Watch TV or read in the bedroom.
Balance activity and rest throughout the day. Eat balanced meals or mini-meals.	Be too active one day and be a slug the next.
Allow yourself a transition period before bedtime. Develop a bedtime ritual.	Exercise close to bedtime (i.e., 2–3 hours before you go to sleep).
Get out of bed if you have not fallen asleep after 20 minutes. Go to another room and do something that is not interesting, stimulating, or exciting for one-half hour.	Stay out of bed longer than 30 minutes if you got up because you could not sleep.

to sleep at night. All of our patients find that going to bed and getting up at a fixed time, even if they have slept poorly the previous night, is helpful over time.

◆ *Avoid naps during the day.* Naps may seem natural when you have not slept well the night before. But they often interfere with sleep at night.

◆ *Get up if you have not fallen asleep after 20 to 30 minutes.* Stay up for 20 minutes in another room doing some rather boring activity (e.g., do not do the crossword or read mysteries). If you feel sleepy, don't allow yourself to fall asleep in a chair. Even if you do not feel sleepy, go back to bed after 30 minutes. If you still do not get sleepy after 20 minutes, repeat this ritual. Remember not to do any "arousing" activities (e.g., television, radio) or to think about worrisome topics when you are up. For the first week or so you may feel somewhat tired during the day, but your body and mind will gradually learn that you mean business when it comes to sleep. Keep with this until you fall asleep for the entire night. Remember, even if you are bone-tired, you cannot force sleep. But you can set up the right conditions for sleep.

◆ *When not asleep in bed at night, relax your muscles.* Even if you do not fall asleep, lying relaxed will help you feel better. If you fall asleep in a relaxed manner, you will feel much more rested. You might find this a good time to review some of your pleasant mental images.

A (Necessary) Return to Pacing

Pacing is so important that although we have covered it in lesson 2, we want to stress it here as well. A pattern of overactivity followed by exhaustion and pain most often leads to poor sleep. For example, if you are overactive one day and underactive the next, the following night you are unlikely to sleep well. The body loves consistent and healthy patterns. (It will get hooked into bad patterns but it really prefers good patterns to follow.) Taking breaks from activity on schedule (rather than when you are exhausted) is a good pattern. Getting up and being active on schedule (rather than when you feel like it) is a good pattern as well. As mentioned earlier, some of our patients buy an inexpensive kitchen timer to remind them when a period of rest or activity is scheduled to occur. This kind of balance gradually builds into a serene and healthy lifestyle that decreases pain and increases enjoyment.

We call this "balanced growth," as illustrated in Figure 4.2. Staying between the dotted lines (optimal level of activity) means growth, success, and energy. Too much activity or inactivity means setbacks, anxiety, failure, and fatigue.

Remember, the pattern of resting before becoming excessively tired is not laziness. It is healthy pacing that allows you to have energy in reserve. During a break from activity, you should plan to do something pleasant and relaxing, something that you enjoy. It's best to determine before your activity period what it is you want to do when you rest.

Regularity is the key to pacing. Skipping a break to try to do more or skipping activity when you want to do nothing often leads to a loss in the ability to be active when you most want to. Moreover, this kind of irregularity can often increase pain and interfere with sleep.

In the beginning, however, it is important to experience success. So choose restful activities and more energetic activities for periods of time that you can handle. Increase these gradually, so that you can be energized by improvement.

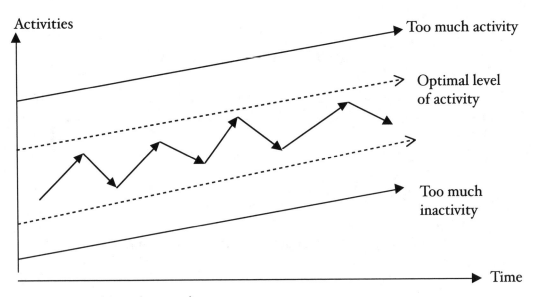

Figure 4.2. Balanced growth.

The Importance of Realistic Expectations in Combating Fatigue

Many of our patients observe that they need to rest for a rather long period after they first start exerting themselves. They consider this to be abnormal ("After all, I'm not 99!"). These thoughts bring up all kinds of distressing feelings—shame, guilt, sadness, frustration. You may feel this as well. What you were able to do in the past (Figure 4.3) was what you considered a decent level of exertion followed by a brief period of rest and recovery.

Your typical day in the past went like this: you woke rested, carried on a number of activities during the day, rested at the end of the day, and finally you went to sleep. This activity–rest cycle most likely became connected to your feelings of success, your sense of self-worth, and your level of confidence. You may not have been aware of this at the time, because you considered it "normal."

When you begin to experience chronic pain, this "normal pattern" may be disrupted entirely or at least in large part. When this occurs, or if you try to push yourself back into your earlier pattern too soon, the result will likely be feelings of failure, loss of self-esteem, and diminished confidence. Nevertheless, old habits die hard. Many of our patients used to

Your old pattern

NORMAL BEARING CAPACITY

14 Hours   10 hours

ACTIVITY		REST

Working, exertion   Relaxing and Sleeping

Self-worth, satisfaction, and confidence

Figure 4.3. Common pattern of activity before chronic pain.

get up each morning resolving to achieve their old activity pattern. In the evening, they feel dejected and as if they have "failed."

These patients, when they first see us, are only able to reach the activity level shown in Figure 4.4.

Is the activity pattern shown in this figure familiar to you? Does it reflect the reality of your life?

If it is, you may find that hard to accept right now. This is okay, too. Acceptance takes time and patience. But it's hard to move from where you are to where you want to go until you begin to accept what has happened as the result of your pain. You may need to grieve these losses in ability to be active in order to accept them and move on.

Part of why people push themselves too hard is that they begin to up their activity level, feel happy and hopeful, and try to immediately return to their earlier levels of activity. For

1–2 hours   22–23 hours

EXERTION	INACTIVITY

Figure 4.4. Chronic pain activity pattern: The new reality.

PACING

1–2 hrs	1–2 hrs	2–3 hrs	1–2 hrs	2–3 hrs	2 hrs	1–2 hrs	Sleep
Exertion	Relax	Exertion	Relax	Exertion	Relax	Exertion	Relax

Typical results: Success, increased self-esteem, and reduced pain

Figure 4.5. The new pattern of activity: A better approach.

these people, acceptance of their current limitations may be one of the most difficult tasks they face in this book. A more appropriate pattern of activity for people who have chronic pain was described in lesson 2. However, acceptance and the level of pacing (see also Figure 4.5) can lead to more consistent days of higher self-esteem, feelings of greater success, and more pain reduction. This is a message of hope to all who suffer from chronic pain

Diversion, Priorities, and Control

Although some of these topics have been or will be discussed in more detail in other lessons, we would like you to consider them here with regard to combating your chronic fatigue.

Diversion

In addition to pacing, the diversion activities described in lesson 3 bear repeating in terms of chronic fatigue and sleep problems. A change of scenery, getting out of a rut, or doing something nice (alone or with others) gives us a boost. Journaling, painting, drawing, sewing, quilting, collecting things, enjoying nature, a weekend away, a good film, an interesting book, and an exciting TV series can all be useful distractions. Beware of perfectionism in some of these more "artistic" pursuits, as this can add stress to your life.

Priorities

When you're in chronic pain, it's easy to lose sight of priorities. But it is helpful to give what attention you can to those things that deserve it—the truly important things in life. For different people, this means different things. For some it means family, for others, it means friends, for still others, it means the ability to pursue some hobby or creative outlet. By *creative outlet* we do not mean painting the Sistine Chapel. Cooking a delicious and beautifully presented meal is creative. Arranging a vase of flowers with mindfulness is creative.

What is important to you now? What has been important to you in the past? What was "worth the trouble" to do before your pain began? Who was it important to stay in contact with? Setting priorities is most important for people with chronic pain and fatigue, because energy is more limited for them than for people without pain.

What are your time-wasters or energy-drainers? Certain people, certain thoughts, mindless television? Dwelling on the past? These all consume precious energy. Prioritize them out of your life

If you are still working inside or out of the home, you may believe that hard and long hours of work are important. But most people realize at least at retirement or at the end of their lives that work has not been that important.

When you ask children, "What do you value most in your parents?" or when you ask adults, "As a child, what did you consider your parents' best attribute?" the answer is never, "They kept the house clean and worked hard at the office." Nor is it, "They worked hard so that we could have lots of money." The answer that is more common in happy families is, "They had time for me." "They showed interest in me." "They listened to me and truly got to know me." These are important things to ponder not only with regard to others but with regard to oneself.

How much of your time is spent showing interest in your whole self, not just your pain? How often do you truly listen to your own heart? How well do you know yourself?

Control

Another energy drainer is trying to control things that are not under your control. On the other hand, if you put your energy into things that you have some control over, with practice (e.g., pacing, nutrition, acceptance, perseverance, patience) you will feel more successful, hopeful, and energetic. Your pain will likely become easier to bear.

Remember the Serenity Prayer: "Grant me the serenity to accept the things I cannot change, the courage to change things I can, and the wisdom to know the difference between the two."

Activities That Can Help

Critical Activities

1. Review the following list of pleasurable activities below and choose five you would like to do and think you could do despite your pain. List these in the spaces provided.

1 _____

2 _____

3 _____

4 _____

5 _____

Now select two from the list you made and put a circle around them. Try one this week and one the next. Record in your journal how tired you felt before and after.

Partial List of Pleasant Activities

1. Spending time outdoors
2. Watching a sporting event
3. Talking to someone about sports
4. Going to a movie
5. Going to a library
6. Going to a museum
7. Planning a short trip.
8. Buying something affordable for yourself or others
9. Looking at relaxing pictures (such as water or nature scenes)
10. Doing something "creative"
11. Reading the Bible or other inspirational literature
12. Reading an engrossing book
13. Playing a few holes of golf
14. Rearranging things in one corner of your house
15. Going to a tavern or other place to socialize
16. Going to a restaurant
17. Going to a lecture
18. Going for a drive in the country
19. Writing poems
20. Knitting or sewing
21. Seeing friends
22. Visiting or being visited by family or friends
23. Having lunch with a family member or friend
24. Spending quiet time with a pet
25. Spending time with your children, grandchildren, nieces, or nephews
26. Going to church
27. Going to a service, civic, or social club

28. Playing a musical instrument
29. Canning, freezing, or making preserves
30. Making food or crafts to give away or sell
31. Playing pool or billiards
32. Playing chess or checkers
33. Playing cards
34. Helping someone else
35. Watching birds or animals
36. Working in your garden
37. Visiting a public garden
38. Going to a zoo or aquarium
39. Listening to the sounds of nature
40. Having a lively conversation with someone
41. Listening to the radio
42. Getting a massage or back rub
43. Going on a picnic or barbecue
44. Buying something for a family member
45. Walking in the woods, mountains, or by the sea or lake
46. Going fishing
47. Going swimming
48. Learning to do something new
49. Talking on the telephone
50. Joining or calling a self-help group such as the American Chronic Pain Association[1]

51. Cooking a meal
52. Writing in a journal
53. Playing a board game (e.g., Monopoly, Scrabble)
54. Playing table tennis
55. Going to a sauna
56. Starting a new project
57. Beginning to work again on an old project
58. Bird-watching
59. People-watching
60. Repairing something
61. Writing letters or postcards
62. Caring for house plants
63. Taking a leisurely walk
64. Collecting something or working on your collection
65. Going to a garage sale
66. Doing brief periods of volunteer work
67. Making a new friend or calling an old one
68. Planning travel with a group
69. Going to a play
70. Teaching something to someone
71. Copying your recipes for others
72. Saying prayers

[1]American Chronic Pain Association telephone number: (800) 533-3231; Web site: http://www.theacpa.org/; e-mail: acpa@pacbel.net

List others that come to your mind.

2. If you are having trouble sleeping, keep a sleep and caffeine diary. Begin by recording the time you go to sleep at night and estimating how long it takes you (approximately) to fall asleep each night. If you nap, write down how many naps you take, when you took them, and how long they lasted. Keep track of the amount and times you consume drinks or food with caffeine. How many times a week do you spend in bed doing activities other than sleep or sexual intimacy? These facts will give you a baseline from which to work.

3. Keep a food diary for 2 days. Record everything you eat including snacks and when you ate them. In your notebook or journal, describe how tired you were before and after eating each meal or snack.

4. Make a list of your top five priorities in life (e.g., grandchildren, finances, hobbies, religion).

Optional Activities

5. Choose a time-consuming task you have been putting off and plan how you can gradually complete this task by pacing over a week or two.

6. Consider the following questions carefully and write down your answer in your notebook or journal: How much acceptance have you experienced with regard to your current limitations? Does acceptance mean that you made your peace with your limitations? How might you begin to accept that your pain and your former way of managing it has caused you difficulty? Would talking to someone about this help?

Don't Let Pain Ruin Your Relationships!

Open yourself genuinely to all people
By being willing to fully communicate your deepest feelings,
Since hiding in any degree keeps you stuck in your illusion
Of separateness from other people.
—Ken Keyes and Bruce Burkan

*A*s you know by now, many people are uninformed about pain. They often assume that pain, although unpleasant, is temporary. They also believe that it will, within a brief time, be easily treated or will simply go away on its own. By extension, they may believe that the person who continually experiences pain is not really feeling pain, is not following doctor's orders, is complaining excessively to get attention, or is trying to avoid some undesirable activity. When people complain of chronic pain, others often consider them weak (or in common parlance, "wimps").

Many of our patients believe that the people around them think one or more of these things. Do you? If you do, you may feel misunderstood, lonely, distressed, frustrated, angry, or some combination of these emotions.

The Importance of Communication

Other people may say well-meaning things, but their words may inadvertently make things worse. "Give it time," one may say. But you have already given it lots of time. "You need to see another doctor," a second suggests. But you have already seen three doctors. "Have you tried ibuprofen?" a third asks. These kinds of suggestions or questions sometimes make you wish that everyone would just leave you alone.

However, there are times you don't want to be left alone. Chronic pain is a lonely experience. You may feel abandoned by others. You may wish for emotional support, especially when the pain is at its worst. And you honestly do need help with some things at some times. If only they knew how hard it was for you to ask!

On their first visit to our offices, many of our patients tell us that their lives now revolve around their bed, lounge chairs, TV, doctors' offices, clinics, and pharmacies. They feel lonely and isolated. Does this describe your situation?

The likelihood of feeling isolated in this situation is greater if you feel you have no one with whom you can freely share your feelings and know that they are not judging you. Perhaps you find it hard to express yourself. Perhaps you attach great value to your independence and don't want to admit that you need support. Or perhaps there is no one around who truly understands.

Your Role in Effective Communication

But first consider this. Friends and family members can feel excluded, powerless, and frustrated if you do not communicate your feelings to them in an open way—a way in which they can truly hear you. If you cannot clearly express your feelings and accurately describe what you need from them, it is hard for them to support you. In all relationships, it is the quality, not the quantity, of communication that determines whether people become distant and defensive or whether bonds are strengthened and deepened. The more people skillfully share each others' lives, each others' desires and longings, each others' worries and uncertainties, the greater their mutual satisfaction. This kind of communication may be difficult for you if you haven't first communicated these things to yourself.

If you can clearly express what you do need and what you do not need, first to yourself and then to others, and if you let family and friends know that they can play a meaningful and important role in your recovery, then you have a real chance at gaining support, affection, and encouragement. Most important, you will not feel so alone. The feelings of safety and security that result make pain easier to bear for everyone. For the person suffering from chronic pain, these feelings reduce stress, help him or her get important needs met, and thus actually can decrease pain. Even when pain is at its worst, feeling safe and secure through trust and understanding makes the pain easier to bear.

In this lesson you will learn about

- ◆ the impact of chronic pain on other people;
- ◆ the importance of good communication and assertiveness;
- ◆ ways to improve your communication and assert yourself; and
- ◆ how to create a supportive environment.

To begin, consider the experience of one of our patients with regard to how chronic pain affected her relationships with other people.

Rita is a 46-year-old woman who has suffered from 3 years of severe and chronic pain following a car accident in which she was rear-ended. She initially suffered from a whiplash injury that was treated. But the pain diminished very little and has now spread from her neck to multiple areas of her body. She has recently been diagnosed with fibromyalgia.

Rita also reports frequent headaches, tingling in her fingers and toes, difficulty sleeping, trouble concentrating, and chronic fatigue, even when she gets a good night's sleep. She reports that almost any activity makes her pain worse.

Rita's pain has been severe enough to disrupt all aspects of her life (work, social, family, and recreational). Her pain does not permit her to get a good night's sleep. Consequently, she never feels rested and is tired most of the time.

Rita acknowledges that since her injuries, she has not had time for her husband, Paul, and her teenage children, Greg and Tara. Her house is no longer as neat and tidy as it used to be.

Paul was initially sympathetic but now says that he is fed up with her constant complaints. The expenses of her medication and medical treatments have drained the family's finances. This has meant giving up family and other pleasurable joint activities. Paul says this wouldn't be so bad, but Rita has no interest in any previously enjoyed activities or even in sex. She just wants to be "left alone."

Rita's children are troubled by her behavior as well. They feel that she has become a different person since the accident. They are anxious about her unpredictable behavior and mood swings. They feel discouraged by her lack of progress toward being "their old mom."

When they are around Rita, they are extremely solicitous, getting her snacks, coffee, medication, and rubbing her neck. Inside, though, they seethe. Rita is uncomfortable asking for things, so she ends up ordering them around. At times, she belittles them for no apparent reason. No matter how well or quickly they do the housework, it never seems to meet her standards. Then they feel they cannot do anything that will please her. They will never be "good enough" for the injured Rita.

At the time Rita and her family come for a consultation with us, the teenagers are confused and angry, and they have begun to stay away from home as much as possible. At the same visit, Rita acknowledges that she is angry with them because they avoid her. She accuses them of not caring. Then she begins to cry, admitting that she feels depressed and guilty about her words and behavior.

Paul, who is a plumbing supplies salesman, has also recently been spending more and more time away from home, often volunteering for extended selling trips. His inaccessibility has led to more anger on Rita's part. The continual conflicts have driven Paul even further away, and he has had some fleeting, but not serious, thoughts about getting a divorce.

Unfortunately, Rita's story is all too common. Living with chronic pain not only causes the patient to suffer but also has an effect on every member of the family.

Are you aware of the impact of your pain on others? Have you noticed how their behavior affects what you think, how you feel, and what you do? What advice would you have for Rita? What would you say to Paul and the children?

Sharing With Family and Friends

There is an old expression, "A sorrow shared is a sorrow halved." Living is sharing both the good times and the bad. The more people share in each other's lives, the greater the likelihood their relationships will bring mutual fulfillment.

When one family member has chronic pain, this kind of sharing and mutual involvement becomes more difficult. Things the couple or family used to do together they can no longer do. Time and money spent on visits to the doctor take the place of time and money for dinners out or nice meals at home.

We tell our patients that first they need to think about how they can compensate for lack of time with their families and friends. We stress the importance of *quality time*. We teach them to use their time together wisely, communicating interest and attention with words and with actions. Many of our patients have closed themselves off from others, however, especially if their pain is long-standing. It takes time and courage to open up again.

How about you? Do you feel that you do not want to "bother" others with your problems? Do you want understanding and support from others but are afraid or embarrassed to have to ask for help? Do you like to give, but have difficulty receiving? When you have done a great deal for others, do you feel especially let down when you get little in return? Do you find yourself being irritable with others, barking orders when you cannot bear to ask for things? Do you act as though all is well and hide your feelings until a final drop causes the bucket to overflow? Does the straw that broke the camel's back lead you to let out all your emotions in one burst?

The answer "yes" to any of these questions is a wall that you may have built to protect yourself. This need to protect yourself is understandable, but you may also be harboring a deep longing for others to break down these walls that you have created. When they don't, you may feel that you have to protect yourself even more.

Your family and friends are likely confused and at times hurt by your behavior (e.g., a sudden outburst of emotion). It is likely that, like Rita, you feel ashamed, confused, and hurt after an outburst as well.

You may then seek to get yourself "back in control" of your feelings. Others may not dare to discuss what has happened. Like you, they try to act as if nothing is wrong. Few people know how to handle so many intense and confused feelings, either in themselves or in others. (Remember how Rita's family responded to her?) Your friends and family may feel as inadequate and helpless as you do at times. They may not know how to respond and how to be supportive.

Most people hope that problems in relationships will disappear on their own. The problem is, they never do. The only way to solve this problem is to learn to communicate better.

Decoding Communication Problems

What are some common problems in communication? Most problems communicating involve the following:

1. *A mismatch between what you say and what you want to say.* For example, saying that you "want everyone to go away" when what you really need is either comfort or just a little bit of time to yourself.
2. *Resistance or confusion about making requests.* You may communicate passively (e.g., through body language) and deny your feelings (even to yourself). Or you may communicate aggressively and defensively, thus hurting others' feelings and not respecting their needs.
3. *Difficulty in active listening to what others are trying to communicate.* You may listen but not really *hear* what is being said.
4. *Making excessive demands, emphasizing dependency, and being dishonest.* Out of frustration, you may regress to a more childlike state in which you expect people to read your mind. When we are in pain, we may think that people close to us *should* understand how we feel, *should* know what we want, or *should* know what to do. When they don't, we may resort to manipulation.

Notice that we have said "you" or "we" throughout. This is because change starts with the person most motivated to change. And that is most likely the person in the most pain—you. Others in your life may have just as much difficulty communicating, but you cannot control them. The only person you can control is yourself.

However, asking why others are not sensitive to your pain is a reasonable question. It may help to think about the following. First, chronic pain is invisible. That is, a person with chronic pain may look quite healthy outwardly but feel miserable on the inside. The inconsistency between appearances and feelings makes communication especially complicated.

For example, as a result of your pain, you may have a number of limitations. This has consequences for other people in your life, who need to know about these. If you "look" fine, other people will automatically assume that your pain is getting better. So, you need to tell them clearly what your limitations are. Particularly in the case of chronic pain, people may need to be told more than once what you are able and not able to do.

Second, people may seem insensitive because it is difficult for them to know what they should or should not do, when to offer help, and when to back off. Men, in particular, may be confused about this. In modern society, most men have been socialized not to notice when others need help. They often do not want to notice when they themselves need help. For example, think of the times a man will drive around lost for an hour before asking for help. Most people assume that he doesn't want to ask for help. But part of the problem is that the man may not even be aware for a while that he needs help.

Third, most people find it difficult to imagine that pain will not end or that it will be a constant companion. Most people are capable of imagining what it means to be dependent on a wheelchair to get around. Those who have difficulty imagining this can spend a day in a wheelchair and they will then know what it's like. (Although it's never really the same, because at the end of the day the person trying out the wheelchair knows that he or she can get up and walk.)

In the case of pain, particularly chronic pain, it's very hard to put yourself in the shoes of another. This is because pain is personal and also because most people's experience with their own pain is with temporary injuries. Unless they have experienced chronic pain, it is truly incomprehensible to them. Other reasons that people may seem to be insensitive to pain include the following.

Other People's Pain Is Not Interesting!

Although you may feel left out of things because of your pain, although some days you wish you could make someone understand exactly what the pain feels like, many people are not naturally predisposed to hearing about this. Although it's very frustrating when the other person doesn't really seem interested in your pain, the hard fact of life is that *pain is NOT that interesting unless it's happening to you!* It helps not to take this personally. When people are uninterested in your pain, it's most often not that they're not interested in you. They likely would not be interested in anyone else's pain either.

Other People Have Their Own Problems

Many people do not wear their hearts on their sleeves. They may be preoccupied with their own problems, but often they do not admit this. Even in a marriage, people may not share their worries. Men, in particular, have often been taught not to talk about a problem until they have it solved. Also, most men have been trained to "solve others' problems" in a concrete way. If they can't fix it, they often don't know what to do. As a result, they may feel inadequate and helpless. Women too, may feel the need to keep a "stiff upper lip" or to try to "fix" things. Most people don't realize that simply listening to another is perhaps the greatest source of comfort there is.

A related issue is that when you share your feelings of sadness, fear, or frustration, they may touch others' feelings of the same sort (e.g., anxiety over financial or work problems, sadness over an elderly parent's ill health). If other people do not want their emotions to be touched by a discussion of yours, they may change the subject. If you continue to talk about your pain or associated emotions, they may remove themselves physically or emotionally from the conversation.

Pain Is a Difficult Subject

People usually like to avoid difficult topics, even if they have nothing negative going on in their own lives, and physical pain is a difficult subject (as is dying, being unemployed, etc.). People may also think if they talk about your pain, it will make things worse. Again, if you continue talking about it, they may tend to back away. But again, this has more to do with them than with you.

Pain Is Not Constant

You likely have noticed that some days your pain is better and other days it is worse. People outside of the home, however, tend to see you when things are going well and not when you are stuck in the house because of the pain. When people see you during a better day, they may quickly assume that you are "better" or that your ongoing pain is "not that bad."

You, on the other hand, know and possibly fear that there will be even worse days ahead, so you may feel a certain reluctance to tell others that you are feeling somewhat better. You are afraid that this will give you as well as your family and friends false hope. These anticipations can influence what you think and feel and do. We will return to this important issue later in this book.

Pain Is Unpredictable

Pain, as you know, does not always follow immediately after overexertion. It can be delayed, which is confusing to other people. They see you being very busy, and then a day or so later you are unable to do much at all. They are not sure what to expect of you. Only after they learn about the ups and downs of living with chronic pain can they understand. However, they may not be ready to learn this until better communication is established between you.

Also, pain makes it difficult to plan ahead. People close to you may feel frustrated because they can never be quite sure what type of day you are likely to have, and they therefore can't plan anything that includes you. People like to give to people they care about, and not being able to plan an outing for you may be as frustrating for them as it is for you.

Pain Causes Negative Feelings

As we have noted pain, fatigue, and limitations all produce negative emotions. Sometimes you give the message, "Help me, don't you see that I'm having a difficult time?" while in an exactly comparable situation you may spitefully say, "Don't help me, let me take care of myself, do you think I can't do anything anymore!" How did Rita feel about her family's responses to her?

As we have illustrated, pain is a complicated topic that is very difficult to understand, not only by you but also by significant people in your life. It is a subject that people would rather avoid.

Improving Communication

Because of these difficulties in understanding chronic pain, learning to communicate well with others is particularly important. Most people have not been trained to communicate well, and most of the time, they "get along" pretty well anyway. However, when difficulties arise, problems in communication make things even worse. So if you have chronic pain, it is important to learn to be an excellent communicator.

To begin this process, we have summarized a few basic guidelines for improving communication in Exhibit 5.1.

Giving and Getting Respect

In addition to these guidelines, it is important to understand the nature of giving and receiving respect. For example, lashing out or engaging in arguments that hurt or anger you or others may damage mutual respect. Expressing yourself *appropriately assertively* is one way to address this problem.

Assertion involves standing up for personal rights and expressing your thoughts, feelings, and beliefs in direct, honest, and appropriate ways. The basic messages when you are communi-

Exhibit 5.1. Guidelines for Improving Communication

✓ Tell others respectfully what you can and cannot do.

✓ Inform them that the severity of your pain varies, even if it is never completely gone.

✓ Tell them in a friendly way what kind of help you hope to receive and why.

✓ Tell them when they are helping! Praise wins over blame every time.

✓ Do not be afraid to tell people when things are a bit better or a bit worse.

✓ Try to be positive, despite the pain. A pleasant disposition can sometimes decrease pain at the same time it brings others closer to you.

✓ Ask for understanding with regard to your difficult feelings about the pain and its consequences. Give a short answer to the question "How are you feeling?" Then show interest by inquiring as to how the other is doing.

✓ Talk to others regularly, not just when your pain is most intense.

✓ Do not have an important discussion, make rash statements, or make important decisions when your pain is at its worst.

✓ Do not use body language to indirectly communicate pain. Be direct and honest in telling people how you are feeling. Encourage others to express their feelings and to discuss them with you.

✓ Do not feel guilty if the pain has a negative influence on your moods; this is normal. Try not to take things out on other people, however.

✓ Work on accepting your present limitations while making efforts to improve.

✓ Do not take the other person's mildly negative behavior personally. Others' moods most often reflect their own personality or concerns.

cating assertively are the following: "this is what I think"; "this is what I feel"; "this is what I would like to happen." These messages express who you are, how you see the problem, and what you want to do about it. If they are communicated appropriately, they do not shame, humiliate, or put you or other people down.

Two types of respect are involved in assertive communication: respect for oneself and respect for the other person. The following is an example of an assertive communication.

A woman was desperately trying to get a flight to Kansas City to see her mother who was sick in the hospital. Weather conditions were bad and the lines were long. Having been rejected from three standby flights, she again found herself in the middle of a long line for the fourth and last flight to Kansas City. This time she approached a man who was standing near the beginning of the line and said, pointing to her place,

"Would you mind exchanging places with me? I ordinarily wouldn't ask, but it's extremely important that I get to Kansas City tonight to be with my mother who is very ill." The man nodded yes.

When asked what her reaction would have been if the man had refused, she replied, "I would have been disappointed but it would have been OK. I hoped he would understand, but after all, he was there first."

In this example the woman showed self-respect by asking whether the man would be willing to help her. Also, she respected the man's right to refuse her request and not fulfill her need.

Assertion, Nonassertion, and Aggression

There are basically three ways to communicate to other people: assertively, nonassertively, and aggressively.

The goal of *assertion* is clear communication and mutuality—to give and receive respect, to play fair, and to leave room for compromise. In the case of compromise, neither person sacrifices the basic integrity of their needs (not wants). Most important, assertion is not simply a way of getting what one wants

Nonassertion involves violating one's own integrity by failing to express honest feelings, thoughts, and beliefs. For example, nonassertion is expressing one's thoughts and feelings in an apologetic, self-effacing manner. It results in others not taking your needs seriously and may reflect that you don't take your needs seriously either.

Nonassertion also sometimes shows a subtle lack of respect for the other person's ability to shoulder some responsibility and to refuse requests appropriately. Ultimately, the goal of nonassertion is to appease others and to avoid conflict.

Aggression involves insisting on one's personal rights in a way that is inappropriate and almost always violates the rights of the other person. The goal of aggression is to dominate and win. Tactics include humiliating and belittling or overpowering people so that they are less able to express and defend their needs and rights

Exhibit 5.2 summarizes the differences between *assertive*, *nonassertive*, and *aggressive* communication.

Behavior as Communication

Your partner or best friend is usually the most important person in your life. He or she is also the one person other than you who is most directly affected by your physical condition. The chronic pain of one's partner or close friend can cause extra strain on a relationship and

Exhibit 5.2. Comparing Nonassertive, Assertive, and Aggressive Behavior

Feelings	Characteristics of the behavior		
	Nonassertive: emotionally dishonest, indirect, self-denying, inhibited	Aggressive: inappropriate, self-enhancing at expense of another	Assertive: appropriate, emotionally honest and direct, self- and other-enhancing, expressive
Your feelings when behaving this way	Hurt, anxious at the time, and possibly angry later	Righteous, superior, maybe feel a sense of relief at the moment, but possibly feel guilty later	Confident, self-respecting, both in the moment and later
The other person's feelings about him or herself when you engage in this behavior	Superior, guilty if they take advantage of your nonassertion	Hurt, humiliated, angry, usually later	Valued and respected
The other person's feelings about you when you engage in this behavior	Pity, irritation, disgust	Angry, vengeful	Generally respectful

communication skills. It's a challenge, and it can cause both people to grow in strength and mutual respect if communication skills are enhanced.

Other people, however, can behave in ways that unknowingly (on their part and possibly on yours) actually have a harmful influence on you. This is true even when they have the best of intentions.

Sometimes your friend may be too understanding and sympathize too much with you (Type A, described below). Sometimes your partner is too afraid to show understanding out of fear that this will make you feel worse (Type B, described below). Just for the sake of understanding, we will portray both types in the most extreme manner. Most people do not fit into "type" this dramatically, but you may recognize some characteristics of each type of person in the family and friends that you have.

Type A Partner or Friend

If your friend is the caring type, he or she may humor you as much as possible and shield you from things that you should be responsible for. They continually take everything out of your hands, believing they are protecting you. If you feel demeaned by this and suddenly get angry or even assert yourself, the Type A friend resignedly accepts your outbursts and may then be condescending.

A Type A friend does not bother you with his or her own problems and instructs others (children, family, friends, neighbors) not to make their problems known to you. They may believe this is helpful "training" so these people will not upset you. When hearing you are in pain, these people will try to get you into bed as quickly as possible. They promptly bring you medication or call the doctor.

A Type A friend may not like others to help you, because they feel that this might be an indication of personal failure on their part. They continually say, "Let me do that." They act as if they very much want you to remain totally dependent on them. Obviously, we have painted an extreme caricature, but some of these characteristics may ring a bell.

Type B Partner or Friend

A Type B friend usually assumes that your pain cannot be as bad as you say. They cannot accept your losses in the areas of daily functioning and your feelings about these losses. They encourage you repeatedly to be strong (subtly suggesting that you are not). They often bring up other people in worse circumstances as examples. "Think about the quadrapalegic who can't even talk without mechanical assistance," they might say. They are also not above using themselves as an example. "I've had pain too, but I didn't let it get me down like you do."

Especially when you want to rest during the day, they are critical. They may directly or indirectly suggest that you are giving in to the pain or, worse, that you are lazy. The Type B person ignores your needs for rest. Particularly when in the company of others, he or she may tell you not be a wimp (or a whiner). The message is loud and clear. You should just tough it out.

When you are feeling upset, the Type B person makes it clear that you should not be so emotional or weak. They often refuse to comfort you when you need it.

Sometimes a person will periodically swing from the Type A to the Type B pattern and back again. This is even more confusing. What is needed is a third type of significant other, a Type C.

Type C Partner or Friend

Type C friends take your pain and your feelings seriously. They talk with you about ways they can or cannot be of help. They don't offer more than they can do, and they assume you will arrange for other help if they're not available. They do not treat you as a patient or as someone "less than" themselves but as an equal person with whom they can share both the good and the bad times in life. The Type C friend does not feel invulnerable to the kind of pain you are experiencing.

This type of person understands that you will experience negative emotions as a result of your chronic pain, but they do not allow you to take it out on them. They express confidence that you can progress in managing your pain, without minimizing the effort involved. They listen and act as a sounding board rather than attempt to solve problems for you.

When they face difficulties, they ask you to listen and be a sounding board as well. They share their own vulnerabilities and limits with you. Please note that this description is just as much of a caricature as our descriptions of Types A and B. Few people behave in a Type C manner in all ways and at all times. They have good and bad days as well.

If you are in a partnership or friendship with someone who is a Type A or B, the most you can hope for is that they will grow and change to become more like Type C at least some of the time. But no one is perfect all of the time. And change, as you well know, takes time and effort.

If your partner or friend is willing, you may wish to ask if they would read this section of the book after you have made a good-faith effort to communicate more effectively. You might use it as a way to begin a dialogue about the pain problem and how it mutually affects you both. Perhaps you may only learn about their feelings. This is okay for now, as long as your partner or friend is not disrespectful. They may have kept things in longer than you have, or they may have enacted their feelings in ways they are not proud of. You can model the patience that you hope they will have with you by accepting them where they are today.

Intimacy

Most people, especially women, but many men as well, know the importance of warm physical contact, especially when one is not feeling well. In any circumstances, such intimacy can help you to be your true self, feel appreciated, and feel safe. Unfortunately, in our society, physical contact can be threatening and may seem less natural than it really is.

Couples in which one partner experiences chronic pain often experience difficulties in the area of sexual intimacy. Sexual intercourse, for example, may be more difficult and less pleasurable as a result of pain and fatigue. Both people may unintentionally avoid physical contact. Also, people often do not have the same needs for physical intimacy at the same time. In the case of sexual intimacy, if one partner longs for tenderness and another for sexual intercourse, unless they understand this, they may reach an impasse.

Fears of failure may disturb the kind of safe atmosphere that both partners need to be sexually intimate. For example, wanting to "perform well" and to give and receive orgasm can disrupt a night of romance. (Outside of physical intimacy, wanting to do well in your own eyes or in the eyes of the other can also seriously disrupt feelings of security and intimacy with the other person. In these cases, you may feel that you are doing something *for* the other instead of *with* him or her.)

It takes really good communication skills to discuss sexuality and negotiate differences in needs for physical contact. A person must feel free to say no to something and to do so in a way that does not hurt the other. This is true in other areas as well. Because pain, tiredness, stress, and uncertainty now play a role in your life, what used to be pleasurable may no longer be so. For example, pain may limit the frequency of the outings you used to go on with a best friend. He or she may not be happy with this and could even be a bit miffed. Feeling free to say no without feeling guilty, even when the other person feels frustrated and takes it personally, is quite a feat. Still, it is vitally important that everyone learns to do this, because doing "yes" and thinking "no" (play-acting) causes tension and may boomerang in other areas of a relationship. Ultimately, it may result in a relationship ending and getting stalled at a superficial level.

Being Romantic

Being romantic may feel like the furthest thing from the mind of a person in pain. But if you make your wishes clear, you may find it relaxing and comforting to be in the intimate company of a person with whom you can be your true self. Being romantic does not necessarily mean being sexual, but it does go beyond friendship. Being romantic may or may not lead to sexual intimacy.

Many people find it romantic to be near a fireplace in winter, to listen to soft music, to have a favorite beverage, to share a favorite film. Others find sharing a big easy chair or comfy couch and holding hands romantic.

What is romantic to one person, however, may not be romantic to the other. One of our patients finds it romantic to wash and dry the dishes with her husband. Her husband feels like this is simply sharing a chore. On the other hand, he feels running errands together is romantic, whereas she feels it is quite stressful. They have to find a mutual ground where both feel relaxed in each other's company and in which closeness can happen naturally.

By itself, warm, safe bodily contact can have a relaxing influence. Tender touch, caressing, nestling safely with each other can all bring feelings of safety and relaxation. It can be a relief (if not necessarily relaxing the first time) when two people try to openly, honestly, and confidentially explain to each other (sometimes with words, sometimes without) what they find relaxing and what they don't when they are together. When there is respect for each other's preferences and values, when there is no shaming, and when communication is open, trust in the other person grows, and clarity and understanding result.

In any relationship, both people need to pay attention to what the other enjoys. Neither person bears responsibility for the quality of the entire relationship. Both must find the time (or make the time) and practice patience in learning to communicate and further intimacy in ways that help the relationship grow.

Relationship Maintenance

Just as a car's engine will burn up if the oil is not changed and replenished, relationships need tune-ups and daily maintenance. These relationship-maintenance steps help both people to act in ways that help the other and create intimacy. Here are some basic maintenance steps to keep in mind:

◆ Remember to balance your immediate needs with the needs of the long-term relationship.
◆ Be gentle when you talk and when you touch.
◆ Be courteous and kind in your actions.
◆ Express frustration and anger directly, with sensitivity to timing. Don't attack or act in a passive–aggressive way.
◆ Don't allow yourself to be threatened, and make no threats to the other person. Be able to tolerate a "no" to requests that you make of another person, and understand that you also have the right to say no.
◆ Try not to judge your significant other when they are not at their best. Perhaps they have reasons completely aside from the relationship for being disagreeable to a request. Avoid thinking (much less saying), "If she loved me she would . . . If he were a good person, he would . . ." Even internal monologues of this sort can bring you down.
◆ Listen and be genuinely interested in the other person's point of view.
◆ Try not to interrupt or talk over the person.
◆ Acknowledge and validate the other person's feelings, wants, and difficulties.
◆ Use appropriate humor to help each other get over the rough spots that occur in any relationship.

While you are reading these suggestions, you might be thinking that it would be great if your significant other would read and heed them. But remember, people change more by example than they do by a lecture. And someone has to start first (usually the most motivated person in the relationship).

Also keep in mind that even when you model these qualities consistently over time, it is unlikely that things will change immediately in your relationship. Troubles in a relationship take time to harden and they take time to melt.

Summary

There is a great deal of ignorance in today's world about the subject of pain, and about chronic pain in particular. Therefore, it may be difficult to find people who automatically understand your situation. The suggestions made in this lesson have the potential to help remedy this situation by helping you understand other people and teaching some of the basics of effective communication. Even if no one but you changes, at the very least you will like looking at yourself in the mirror more if you put some of these suggestions into practice. And the person who looks back at you in the mirror is the person whose opinion of you counts the most.

Activities That Can Help

Critical Activities

1. Covert communication exercise. The following practice exercise may be useful in helping you to describe your pain problem to important family members and friends who may be concerned and possibly confused.

A.   Assume that you are out to dinner with a partner or significant other and you are having a significant increase in pain. Your significant other sees the grimace on your face and asks you what is wrong. What do you say? Write the answer in your journal or notebook.

B.   Identify what it is that you want from this imaginary interaction with your significant other. Would you say this any differently? Do you want your friend to listen, to offer you some reassurance, to offer you some advice, or to offer you some assistance? In your journal or notebook, try rewriting your first sentence to include a clear request for what you may want from the interaction.

C.   What kind of different response do you think that you might get after having rephrased the question to more accurately reflect what you want from the interaction?

2. Refer to the suggestions in Exhibit 5.1 at least once each time you anticipate interacting with other people over a period of a week. Did you see any changes in your behavior or communication style from how you normally behave or communicate? Write down what you noticed in your notebook or journal.

3. How does your partner know that you are in pain? Ask him or her to see if you are on the same page.

4. Arrange a time to discuss your thoughts, feelings, and preferences with someone important to you. It might be best to do this on one of your better days, when your pain is less severe than usual. Write down a day and time to do this here _____. Write down a second date and time (_____) in case you are not able to have this discussion or you feel you should spend more time in this discussion.

How did they react to your request for a discussion? How did the conversation go? How do you feel now that you've had this discussion? Are there other things you would like to say to those close to you? If yes, write them down in your notebook or journal.

5. Complete the assessment listed in Appendix 5.1.

Optional Activities

6. Pick out a difficult situation that recurs in your relationship with someone. Describe the situation and then outline how you might want to express or assert yourself differently in the future and how you might reinforce helpful behavior on the part of the other.

Your difficult situation

DESCRIBE	
EXPRESS	
ASSERT	
REINFORCE	

7. Questions to consider.

- ◆ What do you need most when you are in pain?
- ◆ Is your partner or significant other best described as Type A, Type B, or Type C?
- ◆ Which type do you consider yourself to be?

Appendix 5.1
Pain Rating System

After you have completed the first four critical tasks in this lesson, you will be more than halfway through the program. This will be a good point to return to some of the ratings we included at the end of the first lesson. Please answer each of the questions below. Do not go back and look at your responses you provided after lesson 1. Just make the ratings at this point.

Later, we will suggest you go back and compare your response at different points along the program, but do not go back now. By the end of the program, we expect that you will see changes and improvements. Living with pain is a process, not an outcome. We are confident that with continued effort you will see positive changes occurring in your life.

If you have not already done so, please photocopy the next page, date it, and put it in your journal or notebook.

1. Rate the level of your pain at the **PRESENT MOMENT**.

    0   1   2   3   4   5   6

No pain   Very intense pain

2. In general, during the **PAST WEEK** how much did your pain interfere with daily activities?

    0   1   2   3   4   5   6

No interference   Extreme interference

3. During the **PAST WEEK**, how much has your pain changed the amount of satisfaction or enjoyment you get from taking part in social and recreational activities?

    0   1   2   3   4   5   6

No change   Extreme change

4. On average, how severe has your pain been during the **PAST WEEK**?

    0   1   2   3   4   5   6

Not severe   Extremely severe

5. During the **PAST WEEK**, how well do you feel that you have been able to deal with your problems?

    0   1   2   3   4   5   6

Not at all   Extremely well

6. During the **PAST WEEK**, how successful were you in coping with stressful situations in your life?

    0   1   2   3   4   5   6

Not successful   Extremely successful

7. During the **PAST WEEK**, how irritable have you been?

    0   1   2   3   4   5   6

Not irritable   Extremely irritable

8. During the **PAST WEEK**, how tense or anxious have you been?

    0   1   2   3   4   5   6

Not anxious/tense   Extremely anxious/tense

Changing Behavior

You are more likely to act yourself into feeling
than to feel yourself into action.
—*Jerome Bruner*

Quite naturally, people with chronic pain want to gain control over their pain and their lives. In other words, they don't want to be dependent on their pain. That has been a message repeated throughout this book. But do you really know what it means to be dependent on your pain? You are dependent (i.e., not in control of) on your pain when you allow the amount and severity of your pain to determine

- what you do and how long you do it;
- whether you rest and how long you rest;
- how your mood is;
- whether you take medication and how much;
- whether you ask for help; and
- with whom you socialize.

On the other hand, you can become more independent of your pain if you choose to change your behavior. Knowing what to change and actually doing it are two very different things, as you well know. Often, what we want to do is undermined by habits of which we're not even aware.

To change these patterns, we begin by learning to recognize what factors negatively affect our behavior and what factors are most likely to help us change. We call these the *laws of learning*.

In this lesson, we will show you how your life and your pain are influenced by the attention you give to certain behaviors. Most important, we will show how to change this attention pattern to increase confidence and gain independence from your pain to an extent you never dreamed possible.

Reward Desirable Behavior!

The most important law of learning is that *all behavior is influenced by the consequences of the behavior* (i.e., the results or responses that follow from behavior), whether these consequences are self-induced or are the result of the behavior of others.

Typically, if the consequences are positive, the behavior (good or not so good) will increase and continue. If the results are negative, the behavior will decrease or will not recur. In other words, if you do something and that action is followed by something you like (i.e., a positive reward), it is more likely that you will perform the same or similar actions in the same or similar situations. All of us hope to continue to enjoy positive or desirable outcomes.

If you do something that is followed by something you do not like, you will be less likely to perform the same or similar action again in the same or similar circumstances. You've probably heard the adage "the squeaky wheel always gets the grease." However, you may not be aware of how you are greasing your own squeaky wheels and ignoring the ones that are quiet. That is because most habitual behavior becomes less and less conscious over time. Also, others in your environment may, out of habit, reward undesirable behaviors (i.e., those that keep you stuck) and ignore desirable behaviors (those that could help you become freer). But let's begin by considering a fairly common example that has nothing to do with pain per se but that illustrates these laws of learning.

> Five-year old Katy wants her mother to buy her some new boots with shockingly bright (neon orange and green on black background) colors. Her mother says "No," and explains that these boots do not match her pink coat or that they are too expensive, or she may even say both things.
>
> Katy keeps asking her mother for the boots and refuses to consider any of the other pairs in the store. Her mother repeats her earlier remarks and tells her to select another pair that will better match her coat. Katy now starts to cry loudly, making quite a scene in the store. Her mother tries to soothe and quiet her, but to no avail. Katy's behavior becomes even more extreme, and she finally throws a full-blown temper tantrum. What is it likely her mother will do?

You have likely witnessed such situations or perhaps been in them yourself, either as a child or a parent, grandparent, or guardian. If you were the parent, you may have given in. You were tired, the boots weren't that expensive, and someone was waiting for you. Whatever the circumstances, we have all been guilty of giving in to inappropriate behavior at some point, some of us more so than others.

The important question for our purposes is, if the parent gives in, *What has Katy learned from her experience with the boots?* She has begun to grasp, perhaps even without words, that if she behaves badly in front of others she is more likely to get what she wants. That may not have been the initial intention of her tantrum (she may have been very hungry and tired). But her tantrum produced a desired outcome—she obtained the boots she wanted.

The next time she wants something that her parent is against, she may begin, consciously or unconsciously, to enact the same behavior that won her the boots. If she is successful in this or other attempts to have more power than a little girl should have, the negative behavior will become even more deeply ingrained. Note that we are not saying that Katy is a "bad girl" but that learning experiences are powerful reinforcements of behavior. The more behaviors are reinforced, the more difficult they are to change. Now let's consider the complementary learning lesson—punishing desirable behavior.

Why and how would anyone try to punish (and thereby reduce the frequency of) desirable behavior? No one really does this consciously. However, we do it all the time when we focus on what is wrong and ignore what is right. Another way of putting it is that we pay attention to our own or other's behaviors in a selective fashion. This is a much more difficult-to-undo learning experience, and it occurs whenever desirable behavior may be "expected" and receives no attention. Desirable behavior is, in effect, taken for granted. In the long run, behavior that receives no attention (i.e., behavior that is ignored) often disappears without anyone knowing why.

Again, let's look at a child, this time in his home environment.

Six-year-old Kenny is quietly playing with his toys, and his father is quietly going about his business, either relieved that no more demands are being made of him (he has had a tough day) or perhaps simply not wishing to interfere with his son's age-appropriate play behavior. Kenny's father feels that all is going well. He does not notice Kenny looking up at him from time to time. After a while Kenny gives up on his father and turns on the television.

Kenny's desirable behavior, namely, playing quietly, received no attention or reward from his father. In effect, he was ignored. However, we can by now guess that if he whined, he would likely get some attention, even if it was negative. For children who are feeling ignored, bad attention is better than no attention at all.

Is Kenny's father a bad parent? No. Is he behaving in a way that will increase his son's desirable behavior in the future? The answer here is "no" as well.

Unfortunately, by the time we reach adulthood, we have learned from others not to be attentive to well-running wheels, others' or most especially our own. We tend to enact this behavior with our children.

Attention: A Natural Need

All people need attention, adults as well as children. We especially need the good but taken-for-granted side of ourselves to be "seen" by others, or we will begin to show our other side.

It is human nature to attempt to see ourselves in the eyes of the ones we love, and if we can only see ourselves in their eyes when we practice certain negative behaviors, it is those behaviors that will become patterns in our lives. This occurs most often without conscious awareness.

As a parent, for example, you try to be consistent. You systematically try to reward good behavior and punish bad behavior. But does that actually happen as often as you would like? In the examples of the children Katy and Kenny, you can observe the laws of learning in action. In both cases providing a reward—boots or attention—will likely increase the child's behavior. In Kenny's case, the failure to provide attention (a reward) for positive behavior will likely lead to reduction in appropriate behavior. In these ways, reinforcement can lead to the increase in negative behavior and a decrease in positive behavior.

Let's see how this works with adults, by considering Sandra and Dennis, a married couple.

Dennis likes reading his newspaper and watching TV every night. He only half listens to his wife, Sandra, as she tries to tell him about her day. Without meaning to, his behavior is telling her that what she has to say is less interesting and important than the TV or newspaper. When Sandra asks Dennis to pay attention to her, he either ignores her or behaves as if she is being childish.

Sandra may respond to Dennis's behavior in several ways. She may grumble under her breath, she may get angry outwardly, or she may unconsciously forget to give him an important telephone message. She may not be aware of any of these responses or she may be aware of some.

Assume that none of Sandra' efforts are successful, and Dennis continues to be unresponsive to her efforts to gain his attention. In desperation, Sandra announces that she wants a divorce and begins packing her bags. Suddenly, she has Dennis's attention.

Dennis does not want a divorce. He changes immediately, and suddenly he is ready to give Sandra his undivided attention. He promises to read less and to pay more attention to Sandra, and he brings her flowers the next day.

What has Sandra learned from this experience? She observes that only when she takes extreme measures (not quite tantrums, as in the example of Katy, but the result is the same) will Dennis respond in the way she wishes. Packing her bags was followed by the desired outcome (Dennis's undivided attention). Remember, behavior that produces a desirable outcome will be repeated—a basic law of learning. What do you think Sandra will be likely to do the next time Dennis is inattentive? Now let's consider another example.

Don hurt his back on the job several years ago. His severe pain has affected all parts of his life. He mostly sits in his lounge chair watching TV during the day and stays in bed watching TV at night. He visited a physical therapist who developed an exercise plan for him, making use of the principles of pacing. But every time Don tried the exercises he felt that his pain became worse, and he feared that the exercises recommended would cause more serious damage to his back.

So whenever he started to be active, he used the first sign of pain to lie down. When he did, his pain seemed somewhat reduced.

This example shows how we can produce what we think are "desirable outcomes" by ourselves. What has Don learned from his experience? Several things: "If it hurts, don't do it"; "Exercise causes pain, so don't do it"; and, "If I stop exercising and lie down, my pain is relieved. So stop at any sign of pain."

He has also come to associate activity with pain. Now, even if physical therapy is mentioned, his back starts to act up. It is like the famous dog that Pavlov taught to salivate at the sound of a bell because that sound was previously associated with getting fed. Pavlov's dog wasn't neurotic. He had simply learned to anticipate and to expect food when he heard a bell. Then even when no food was actually present and the light came on, he salivated. The dog and Don learned to expect something to happen on the basis of previous learning.

What impact do you think Don's experience will have on his general behavior? As you might expect, he will become more and more inactive. The more he is inactive, the more he loses muscle strength, flexibility, and endurance. Thus, another vicious circle is created.

Learning to avoid something, like activity, to prevent an undesired outcome is referred to as *the law of avoidance learning*. It is a variant of the first law of learning (i.e., that all behavior is influenced by the consequences of that behavior). In the case of chronic pain, learning to anticipate undesired outcomes (e.g., pain) will cause one to avoid healthy behavior (e.g., staying active).

Exhibit 6.1 summarizes behavior based on both laws of learning presented in this lesson in case examples. Rewards are considered positive reinforcement, whereas undesired outcomes are considered negative reinforcement.

Exhibit 6.1. Case Examples and Laws of Learning

Behavior	Consequence	Reinforcement	Result
Katy—tantrum	Giving in	Positive	More tantrums
Kenny—quietly playing	No attention; neglect	No reinforcement	No longer playing
Sandra—asking	No attention; ridicule	No reinforcement	No longer asking
Sandra—packing	Much attention	Positive	More extreme behavior
Don—exercising	More pain and worry	Negative	No more exercising
Don—lying down	Less pain and worry	Positive	More resting

The Laws of Learning and You

How does attention work in day-to-day relationships? On the positive side, when we look for the good characteristics in others and give attention to these positive elements in our relationships, these relationships will steadily become stronger and closer. That's what tends to happen when one rewards the positive behaviors in relationships by giving them more attention.

On the other hand, if we are continually busy discovering faults in others (our partner, colleagues, boss, or children) and if we criticize or attack others frequently, we negatively reinforce their experience of being around us. Thus, if we reward negative behavior by giving it attention, we'll find that our relationships gradually or rapidly become less satisfying.

For some people, complaints of pain get more and more attention, and this attention influences their behavior in a negative way. For others, feeling pain and maintaining a positive disposition may well be ignored (remember how the squeaky wheel gets the grease). Therefore, people who didn't complain at first about their pain may begin to talk about it or show more and more nonverbal signs of suffering.

This illustrates a principle that was learned when scientists studied abused children. Negative attention is experienced as better than no attention at all. That is part of why abused children often want to return to their homes after they are in foster care. In foster care, where there are many children, they are often ignored. At home, at least they got attention, even if it was painful.

We were all little children once, and we still need attention as adults. Negative attention may be unpleasant, but when we receive no attention, we feel as if we might wither and die. That's why it's natural, although counterproductive, for an adult to seek attention through talking and complaining about pain. The key is to try to find ways to receive needed attention without reinforcing one's own sense of suffering and perhaps driving others away.

By way of review, we have summarized the behavioral principles behind the laws of learning in Exhibit 6.2

Inappropriate Attention

We have seen that attention has a strong power to influence behavior. But specifically, what kinds of attention are desirable and undesirable when it comes to chronic pain? Is it good to give your pain as much attention as possible, or is it better to ignore it? You may be surprised by the answers.

Exhibit 6.2. Summary of the Laws of Learning

Schedule	Consequences	Probability of the behavior recurring
Positive reinforcement	Reward the behavior	More likely
Negative reinforcement	Prevent or withdraw, avoidance	More likely
Punishment	With negative emotions and much attention	More likely
Punishment	With little attention, ignoring the behavior	Less likely
Neglect	Prevent or withdraw positive results	Less likely

Doctor Shopping

Doctors often unwittingly reinforce pain by paying particular attention to increased reporting of pain. The more pain reported, the more attention they give to the patient. The opposite is also true. When people report a reduction of pain, they often receive less attention from their physician. This may have unfortunate results.

When a doctor or therapy no longer provides attention, patients may begin to think about repeating diagnostic tests or searching out new therapies or physicians. Pinning one's hopes on a physician or treatment is natural in the beginning. It decreases feelings of aloneness and engenders hope. However, although new doctors or new treatments may generate hope at first, they may then lead to deeper feelings of hopelessness or a frantic search for other options as relief of chronic pain is not realized. Continued doctor and treatment shopping will eventually bring about increasingly more despair because false hopes and attention will not in themselves reduce pain.

On the other hand, some people with chronic pain stay with the same physician, but they become dependent on him or her for too long a time. This results in a fearful dependence and uncertainty, often followed by lack of hope, frustration, and distress. If the distress brings about attention at that point, they may receive a lot of negative reinforcement for emphasizing their pain.

Only the right kind of attention can take one's mind off pain and focus it toward more productive areas. Think about your own experiences. How many specialists have you sought out? How many medications, treatments, and surgeries have you received? How did you feel when a new treatment was recommended? If your hopes were dashed, how did you feel?

Endless searching for "something new" will also interfere with attempts at self-management of pain. For example, many products and treatments hold out promises of relief. But do their sponsors have any real evidence to back up their claims? We're not talking about personal testimonials or advertisements, but clear scientific proof. Not 9 out of 10 doctors, but real data. Searching after unproven treatments takes time away from learning proven methods that are helpful in reducing both pain and distress and in leading to a better life.

At some point, all of us must accept ownership of our lives. If you have gotten this far in the book, you have begun this journey with regard to your pain. Over time, you will see the benefits in your experience of pain, in your ability to enjoy activities, and in your relationships with other people.

Trying to Fool All of the People All of the Time

Some people try to hide the pain. They think that hiding the pain causes less suffering to those around them. After all, putting on a false positive face may reduce unwanted questions and undesired attention. Too much attention may become annoying and painful itself.

However, the idea that it is helpful to hide the pain all the time is incorrect. Denying a part of reality (the pain) means that you continually have to play a false role, that you continually have to walk on eggshells—in short, that you can never be yourself. Covering up takes a lot of energy. Trying to fool all the people all of the time is exhausting.

But wait a minute, you might say! Wasn't the first part of this lesson devoted to the hidden costs of bringing others' attention to your pain? Yes, that is true. That is where our emphasis was. But you may remember that we also discussed the benefits of sharing, open and honest communication, and obtaining and giving the right kind and amount of attention.

First, you need some attention with regard to your suffering. Without some validation of your pain by someone or by not allowing yourself to receive appropriate attention, you may actually be spending more of your own attention on your pain. This then accentuates your experience of pain.

What is needed is to be honestly open about your pain and limitations with appropriate people at appropriate times. That is, you need to let the *right someone* in on what you are truly experiencing, someone with whom you can be your real self. If you have no one in your life at this time who fits that bill, share your feelings with God, a higher power, or even the "benign universe."

Accentuating the Negative

As we discussed before, the squeaky wheels in our lives get the grease, not only from others but, more important, from ourselves. This is partly because when things are going well, we quickly consider the positive to be normal. Anything outside of this automatically receives our attention.

Remember a time when you had a bad cold. For a few days after the cold had passed, you felt grateful for the fact that you could breathe normally, that your nose wasn't raw, and that your chest didn't feel tight. You felt grateful to be able to do all the normal things that you took for granted. After a while, however, you forgot what it was like to have a cold, and breathing easily felt normal again.

Chronic pain, by its very nature, does not go away like a cold. So it is easy to get stuck on focusing on the negative—the pain. This naturally leads to negative thoughts and emotions. We are not telling you to deny your pain. What we are saying is that if you give it more attention than it is due, you end up paying a double price for your pain. You not only have the pain you started out with, but now you have more negative emotions, more negative thoughts, and an intensified experience of pain.

Think for a moment about all of the distressing emotions humans can feel: anger, fear, depression, shame, guilt, jealousy, sadness, embarrassment, and annoyance, to name just a few. Now, think for a moment of all the pleasurable emotions humans can feel. Were you able to come up with as many? Most people, when asked to think about it, can name more negative emotions than positive ones. It takes work to focus on positive emotions

Think again about your body. When it was functioning properly, you may have hardly given it a thought. Most healthy people do not pay much attention to their bodies unless they are trying to lose weight or are temporarily ill.

Acknowledge to yourself not only when you are in pain but also when you have a good day or even when you feel just a bit better in one part of your body. Try to appreciate this and whatever other positive emotions you may feel. On good days (and on very bad days) try focusing on what you can do or what you have, such as moving more easily or having a varied daily schedule. Try to focus on the small things—a smile from the mailman or a phone call from a friend.

And don't be afraid to admit to yourself when you feel better, physically or emotionally. It will not "jinx" your improvement. It won't give you false hope unless you tell yourself that "now, I'm well for good." As in most things, it's best to take one day at a time.

On bad days, you may want to focus more on the parts of your body that function well, quietly stimulating and activating them. This can start a cycle of feeling a bit better, leading to more pleasant emotions and positive behaviors and feeling even better. On any day (good or bad), you can focus on the healthy parts of your body, perhaps using the relaxation exercises described in lesson 3. These areas of your body deserve as much of your attention as your pain.

Appropriate Attention

You now know that when you pay attention to positive (healthy) behavior, that act is already a positive step. What's important next is to recognize the ways in which you can use your attention effectively as a reward to achieve positive results for yourself and for others.

Four factors determine the effectiveness of any reward: *desirability* (how positive the reward is to you or another person), *timing* (how close the reward is to the behavior that is to be reinforced), *frequency* (how often), and *predictability*. The reward is most effective if it is (a) something that is desired by you or someone else, (b) provided as soon as possible after the desirable behavior, (c) given frequently, and (d) timed in an unpredictable way.

Desired Rewards

Whatever the reward is, it must be viewed favorably by the person to whom it is directed. For example, if you gave someone a box of candy as a reward and they were on a diet, the reward might not be desired. In the case of pain, someone who tells you to take it easy because you do not "look good today" might not be rewarding you if you are trying to do more and to build up your strength. To be positive, the reward, whether attention or some tangible object, needs to be something that the recipient wishes to receive. The more desirable it is, the more motivating.

Prompt Rewards

The reward is most effective if it follows the behavior to be reinforced closely in time. This may be more apparent if we use alcohol and the potential alcoholic to illustrate.

The potential alcoholic individual taking his or her first drink often experiences a reduction in anxiety and worry and an increase in relaxation and sociability as a result of the alcohol. Drinking is thus immediately positively rewarded by these desirable feelings. In fact, anticipating these positive feelings may lead to drinking the next day and the day after that. If a person becomes an alcoholic, he or she may experience many negative consequences later on in the disease process (e.g., loss of job, family, prestige). However, the initial feeling of pleasure that is reinforced soon after a drink may be much more influential than these negative consequences in determining how difficult it is for the alcoholic to quit.

When people with alcoholism are sober, they may be very aware of the losses involved in their disease process and may feel miserable, guilty, and ashamed. Also, when sober, the alcoholic person may feel that people and situations in his or her environment are punishing, therefore negatively reinforcing the state of being sober. However, as soon as he or she takes a drink, these undesirable emotions and punishments seem to fade away. Problems are soon forgotten, and only the present state of alcoholic relief counts—not yesterday and certainly not tomorrow.

The same can be true for chronic pain. You may feel relatively worthless one day because you have done so little, according to your standards. Then, you feel somewhat better the next day, so you overdo it to make up for the "perceived lack" in yourself yesterday. During the activity you may feel fairly well. You taste the satisfaction of being occupied, there is diversion, and there is often a visible result. You feel somewhat better about yourself as a result. So, what's the catch?

The catch is that you are not punished immediately for doing too much, or for doing it too long. The pain typically comes later, the next day or the day after that. It is only then that you discover that you have gone beyond your limitations. The link between behavior and punishment is too far apart in time to be helpful.

Progressing too fast in your activity plan or staying active until you are in pain and are fatigued will feel like a delayed sunburn after enjoying the sun. Or more subtly, if you stop your activities and rest after a certain amount of pain, then *rest* will be the inadvertent reward that follows a certain level of pain. Strangely enough, this will cause that pain level to occur earlier and more often. This is because something good only happens when you feel the pain is extreme, namely, the body receives rest and/or medication. If prescription painkillers are used, then this can surely be a *reward* for experiencing pain.

Along the same lines, perhaps you are only able to ask for attention and help when you feel the pain forces you to do so. In this manner you will become steadily more dependent on severe pain to give you the opportunity to ask for help or to get needed attention.

Maybe you think, "I'm a real fighter. I don't complain and I don't give up quickly. I continue until I can't go on any more. I only stop if the pain and tiredness force me to. I only take medicines when I really can't stand the pain and need them."

If you only rest and take appropriate medicines when you absolutely need to, then you are setting yourself up for failure. Like the alcoholic who only drinks when he or she "needs to," you may be striding straight toward dependence on pain to bring you needed relief.

So with regard to medication, if your doctor has prescribed pain medication and you have pain most of the time, it is usually best to take it at regular times each day rather than only when your pain is at its worst. If you take pain medication only when your pain is at its worst, you inadvertently reinforce that medication is a positive reward for pain. This may actually increase the amount of pain you feel!

In summary, pain medication, rest, and attention should not be directly linked to a certain amount of pain. You should get rest, attention, and help even when your pain is less severe.

Frequent Rewards

Small rewards given frequently tend to work better than a large reward promised in the distant future. Using a parent–child example again to illustrate, sometimes parents promise their child at the beginning of the new school year that they will buy them a much-desired bicycle or computer game if they get all *A*s at the end of the semester. The parents are usually surprised to see that for most children, this incentive has little to no influence at all on daily study behavior. Smaller but more frequent rewards tend to be more motivating for consistent study behavior (e.g., going to the movies or receiving a small amount of money or a small toy at the end of the week). Then, the reward will be closer in time, more frequent, and more linked to the efforts made during the week.

You, too, can only move forward by gradual but persistent effort and a willingness to stick with your self-management plan. Give yourself special attention or rewards for your efforts frequently, even when you don't see objective evidence of "success." In the same vein, try not to dwell for too long on inevitable setbacks. (Some setbacks are to be expected. Most successful nonsmokers tried at least three times before they succeeded in quitting smoking for good.) Remember, you learned to walk and to ride a bike only by falling down and getting up again.

In short, you can have long-term goals, but progress will come more quickly if you strive toward limited goals over the short term and reinforce effort and small successes along the way to longer term goals. It also helps if your partner and other significant people in your life understand your self-management plan and provide encouragement and positive support for your efforts and small successes. It would probably also be best if they paid little attention to any setbacks that naturally occur. We stress this because too often our patients become critical of themselves when they have not achieved their long-term goals as soon as they thought they would.

Keeping the kind of progress charts we described in lesson 2 can provide you with immediate feedback on your *efforts.* Over time, you can see where you started and where you are now. For example, you can see that you started being able to walk 5 minutes and now you can walk 12 minutes. This is success! Perhaps you used to be active around the house 10 minutes three times a day, and now you are active 20 minutes three times a day. This is success! Most important, however, you will see how you have been active in taking charge of your pain and your life.

Unpredictable Rewards

Probably the most surprising thing you will read in this lesson is that rewards are most effective when they are not totally predictable. As mentioned earlier, regular gamblers get "hooked" because they are rewarded in an unpredictable manner (e.g., "One more try on this slot machine and I'll win."). One factor that may account for the appeal of fishing is that is that you do not know exactly when or if you are going to catch a fish. Even presents that are unexpected tend to be more appreciated than predictable presents on fixed dates. This is also true in a relationship. One couple we know gives each other unexpected presents throughout the year instead of on birthdays and Christmas. They then enjoy the birthdays and holidays without the tension that sometimes surrounds these occasions.

Remember the example of Dennis and Sandra earlier in this lesson? What we did not mention is that after learning that Sandra needed positive attention, Dennis started to bring her flowers every Friday. At first, Sandra was delighted. Over time, however, bringing flowers on Friday became routine. Sandra would even forget to notice that that Dennis had brought flowers home. The predictability of the reward had led to it being less rewarding. Now, anyone who's been in a relationship knows that if Dennis stopped bringing Sandra flowers, she would likely be hurt. Perhaps a fight would ensue. At the very least, Dennis would likely hear, in an obvious or subtle accusatory voice, "Why didn't you bring any flowers?"

Thus, failure to do what comes to be expected often creates problems in a relationship. However, a certain amount of unpredictability is desirable, not only in our daily lives but also in our relationships. It is true that a certain amount of predictability provides comfort and order. But progress and other good things in life need surprise rewards; otherwise they have a tendency to disappear.

If you have raised children, you may have learned (or are learning) that unpredictable rewarding of *undesirable* behavior makes this behavior the most stubborn and difficult to change. If a child misbehaves and sometimes you give him or her a time-out and sometimes you don't, the misbehavior is likely to continue and increase in frequency. The unpredictable nature of pain often causes people with chronic pain to gamble with their activity and rest routines. They may even rely on "Lady Luck." One day they feel well, so they think they are lucky and do a lot. A day or two later, they feel bad and rest all day, thinking, "Tomorrow I may be lucky again." In the world of pain, however, gambling in this way only leads to loss.

Preparing for Behavioral Change

As people with chronic pain begin to consider behavioral changes, one problem they often face is that some of their previous behaviors were "rewarding" in the short term. That is, passivity, avoidance behavior, sleeping pills, and so on provided immediate rewards, so it was easy to become hooked on these illusory charms. These rewards may even continue to periodically occur over the long term because of what is known as the *placebo effect*—the mind thinks the unhealthy actions or inactions are working (even when they are not), and so the person is tricked into thinking he or she feels better as a result.

The second problem you may face as you begin to change your behavior is that you may feel "punished" almost immediately. Everyone feels a degree of discomfort or distress when he or she first begins to change (whether this be activity–rest cycles, relationship changes, or dietary changes). You will likely feel this, too, at first. We ask that you persevere *consistently* for at least 6 weeks. Research has shown that it takes consistent change for 6 weeks before people (a) see progress and (b) feel natural with regard to the change. Our patients have taught us that the distress or discomfort felt in the beginning of change is heavily outweighed by the rewards of consistency over time. They also have told us that they could tolerate a lot of discomfort at first when they believed that it would ultimately lead to less pain, less frequency of pain, and more enjoyment of life. Chronic pain is generally purposeless and makes people feel hopeless, because it serves no goal. If you learn to accept and to manage your pain in the ways we have described, you have a goal and a means of reaching that goal, one day and one step at a time. One of our patients summed this up nicely, "I used to feel controlled by my pain, but now I feel I'm in charge of my life, even though I still experience some pain!" This person has overcome her fears, her felt lack of control, and her hopelessness. You can, too!

Summary

Dependence on pain occurs when pain is the driver and you are in the back seat. When you get in the front seat and put pain in its proper place (i.e., the back seat and eventually the trunk), you will begin to feel like life is worth living again. The laws of learning combined with the other lessons in this book can be your driver's manual, helping you to reclaim your rightful place and enjoy a fulfilling life again.

As a recap of this rather complicated lesson, we summarize the main points below.

◆ Reward desirable behavior. This is the most important learning principle. Behavior that is rewarded positively will occur more frequently. Attention is one of the most important and strongest reinforcers of behavior.
◆ Don't reward undesirable behavior. (You know which behaviors are undesirable for you.)
◆ Reward desirable behavior promptly and frequently. If possible, ask someone else to reward your efforts on an unpredictable schedule.
◆ Keep your eye on your long-term goals, but chart progress as effort rather than immediate results. Important changes do not always result in immediate success. Investment in the future is necessary.

Activities That Can Help

Critical Activities

1. List at least three things that you can do for yourself that you would find rewarding. Use these after you have put in effort in your pain management program.

2. Over a couple of days, notice only your positive behaviors, pay attention to them, and dwell on them. Ignore as much as possible negative behaviors. How does this feel?

3. Over a day or two, keep track of the number of complimentary and the number of critical statements you make to people who are important to you. Do the results surprise you and perhaps indicate a need for change on your part?

4. Every day for the next week try to give at least one person a sincere compliment. Notice how they react. Notice how you feel afterwards.

Optional Activities

5. What behaviors would you like to pay more attention to and what behaviors would you like to deemphasize now that you are familiar with the principles of learning?

6. Pay attention to how people respond to you when you tell them you are having a good day or are feeling somewhat less pain.

   a. Do they ignore you?
   b. Do they immediately give you more responsibilities or unrewarding tasks to do?
   c. Do they seem less willing to spend time with you, because you appear "better"? Are they glad that they can go their own way again?

How does this contrast with how they respond when you tell them you are having a bad day or things are not going well?

   a. Do they give you more attention?
   b. Do they spend more time with you?
   c. Do they get frustrated or angry?

If they give you less attention when you are well and feeling good, does this sometimes lead you to try to convince them of the severity of your pain? Can you see a vicious circle here?

7. Keep a reward journal for your efforts for the next 2 weeks. Record your positive behavior (e.g., effort, action), how you rewarded yourself, and how you felt after the reward.

Day	Effort, action	Reward	Feeling after

Changing Thoughts and Feelings

If you are distressed by anything external,
the pain is not due to the thing, but your estimate of it.
This you have the power to revoke at any time.
—Marcus Aurelius

*T*hinking is the way we talk to ourselves (i.e., *self-talk*). Feeling is the way our emotions react to our thoughts or behavior. Thinking and feeling are very different than doing, of course. When our patients are having difficulty with our program thus far, we focus more closely on their thinking and feeling.

Perhaps you may be thinking at this point, "I am practicing the principles of pacing, balance, and learning. I know what I must do to succeed. How come I don't feel better yet? In fact, today I feel lousy."

Although natural at this point, this is the kind of self-talk that can be discouraging and can lead to setbacks in your progress. This is because thoughts and feelings play a central role in continuing to change and experiencing satisfaction with change.

In this lesson you will learn methods that will enable you to influence your thoughts and feelings and, thereby, your pain. These include methods that will help you think more realistically and prevent your feelings from dictating your behavior. If you are having trouble so far and you have been doing all of the critical activities in the previous lessons, these methods may be the key to your breakthrough.

Method 1: Thinking Differently

Try to recall a serious conflict that you have had with someone. What feelings or emotions can you recall before, during, or after this conflict? Did you feel anger, frustration, sadness, or worry? We would like you to consider that you thought yourself into these feelings. And we would also like you to consider that these feelings then influenced the way you later thought and then how you felt—yet another vicious circle.

One major way our habitual manner of thinking gets in our way is that our "interpretation" of problems changes the way we view reality. This distortion leads to feelings that are distressing. And these distressing emotions produce major negative changes in our bodies and hence in our experience of pain.

Our feelings also influence how we think. If we feel upset, we may think, "I really didn't handle that very well. I'm not good at dealing with conflicts." Or, "He is being really mean. I should never have married him."

A second way that distressing feelings from conflicts are intensified is that we think or feel about the conflict or our feelings too much and from only one (typically our own) perspective. This may lead to actions we regret and the negative emotions that follow those actions. We may lash out. Or we may get stuck in feeling sorry for ourselves.

Think of a time when you had a conflict with someone, something that got your mind and emotions all riled up. Then, unexpectedly, something else important and engrossing came up and you were distracted for a day or two. During that period, you probably did not have time to think about the conflict that was so much on your mind before. Likely, the very first time you again revisited the conflict you felt much less distressed. However, if then you continued to dwell on it, you likely aroused the feelings that were put aside. You actually thought yourself into the same spot you were in before you were distracted.

Thinking and feeling are powerful. They can be used to distress us, but they also can be used to help us. For example, just as it is possible to evoke negative thinking and distressing emotions, it is also possible to influence thinking and feeling positively.

In this regard, one of the real differences between a pessimist and an optimist is that the optimist focuses thoughts and feelings on pleasant things, whereas the pessimist focuses on the things that can and do go wrong. For someone thinking pessimistically, even the most positive situation can be viewed negatively.

For example, imagine a pleasant scene in which a couple is having a picnic on a lovely spring afternoon. They are sitting under a tree next to a small brook. Now, in this instance, the wife sees only the positive characteristics of this scene, whereas the husband sees something quite different. She thinks about the beautiful blue sky, the shade the tree is providing, and the delicious meal to come. He, on the other hand, is thinking about the possibility that the grass might stain their clothes, that the food might get infested with ants, that the clouds in the distance portend a storm. As he thinks about these things more and more, he begins to believe that the storm he has conjured up may involve thunder, and they are sitting under a tree. He begins looking at his watch to see if they have enough time to eat before the storm arrives. Who do you think is enjoying their time more?

"Now," perhaps you are thinking, "that's all well and good for a picnic, but what about my pain? That's no picnic at all." That is true, but on a given day, how you think about your pain will influence how you think about other things that day, what emotions you experience that day, how you behave that day, and even how much pain you will experience that day.

For example, perhaps you wake up in pain and begin thinking about how hopeless your situation is, how helpless you feel to influence the pain, and how your friends are off doing things that you cannot do. This leads to your noticing how much the walls need painting, how you can no longer paint the way you used to, and how you can't even have company in because the walls are dingy. As a result of these thoughts, you are likely going to feel sad, depressed, envious, angry, or some combination of these emotions. This, in turn, will increase tension in your body and your sense of exhaustion, and both of these will add to your pain and to your experience of the intensity of your pain. (Remember, your feelings can open the pain gate and make your pain even more intense.)

Negative and distressing thoughts also have the effect of increasing distressing feelings because they lead to focusing on the "worst possibility" in the future (e.g., your whole house is falling down). This soon grows to a probability, and you are likely to end up feeling like a helpless and hopeless captive of your pain forevermore. These thoughts and feelings cause your body to go into "fight or flight" mode (anger, tension) or into complete passivity (depression). Either way, you lose, and your pain increases. Pain seems to be a cruel judge, and you will soon feel as if you have a life sentence without possibility of parole.

"Wait," you may think, "I'm a realist, not a pessimist." But there is a difference between "negative" thinking and "realistic thinking." In Exhibit 7.1, we list some of the negative thoughts our patients have admitted to having. Do any of them sound familiar?

Exhibit 7.1. Negative Thinking

◆ "My pain is terrible!"
◆ "I can't bear it! How long must this go on?"
◆ "I shouldn't have so much pain. I don't deserve this."
◆ "I simply have to find some relief now!"
◆ "Why can't they make my pain go away?"
◆ "I'm going crazy! Where will this all end?"
◆ "I'm going to be an invalid. I can hardly do anything any more."
◆ "I'm a burden to those around me."
◆ "I'll never get better."
◆ "This is going to get worse and worse. Maybe I'll go crazy."
◆ "No one else can ever really understand this pain."
◆ "I'll never be able to enjoy life again."
◆ "It's all my fault that I'm in this mess."
◆ "It's all _____ (my boss's, etc., fill in the blanks) fault that I'm in this mess."

Exhibit 7.2. Realistic Thinking

◆ "The extreme pain is back again, but I know that it is only temporary."

◆ "By relaxing my muscles I can make my pain more bearable."

◆ "I can take a bit more rest today between activities. Tomorrow I'll get back on my regular activity routine again."

◆ "I want to do something pleasant or telephone somebody, as a distraction."

◆ "I can keep my breathing as deep and even as possible and this will reduce my experience of pain."

◆ "Bad days are to be expected, we all have them. I might as well enjoy what there is to enjoy, even on the bad days."

◆ "I can stay in control of the rest of my life, even when my neck hurts."

◆ "Things are going slowly but in the right direction. I'm going to get better and better."

After working the program outlined in this book, these same people learned to think more realistically. Exhibit 7.2 lists their thoughts later on.

Note that the statements listed in Exhibit 7.2 do not indicate that the person's pain is totally gone. Some of them indicate our patient is having a bad pain day. But their realistic thoughts have a much more positive influence on their experience of pain than their negative or pessimistic thoughts, which open the pain gate.

As another example, let's imagine that two different people wake up with a splitting headache. One thinks, "This is a result of that busy day yesterday. I overdid it when I was exercising. I'll take a hot shower and take it easier today." The other thinks, "This is the same pain my father described just before he had that stroke. I'm probably going to have a stroke. I must go to see the doctor immediately. But it is Saturday. What am I going to do?"

The first person now feels more relaxed, less distressed, and more in control. The second person feels anxious, discouraged, and helpless (i.e., dependent on others to feel better). As a result, for the second person, the headache may worsen. By the time the second person gets to the doctor, he will alarm the doctor to the point that she orders a CAT scan. Waiting for the test results, he feels even more anxious and his pain is almost unbearable. Fortunately, the CAT scan shows nothing abnormal. Unfortunately, the relief he now feels reinforces the unhelpful chain of thoughts, emotions and behaviors (i.e., relief is a reward for negative behavior). Both people had a headache, but their reactions resulted in very different consequences.

Here are some more common thinking errors our patients have shared with us:

1. Blaming: They make someone or something else responsible for their pain. "My lousy boss caused my job accident." "My family demands so much from me. That's why I can't afford the time or money to take care of this pain." Or, the blame is turned inward: "It's all my fault that this happened to me." "If only I hadn't . . ."

2. "Should" Statements: The words *should, must,* or *ought* appear regularly in negative thinking and irrational thoughts about pain. "Shoulds" are secret put-downs, implying that a person is stupid, foolish or weak. "I should have thought of good body mechanics before I lifted that box." "I shouldn't have been in such a hurry. That's why I slipped on the ice." "I must keep up with all my responsibilities, pain or no pain." "I shouldn't react to pain like this."

3. Polarized Thinking: Everything is "black or white," "good or bad" when we think in a polarized way. There is no gray area in which reality or improvement can be seen. Polarized thinking is often couched in terms of absolute statements with certain cue words such as *all, every, none, never, always, everybody,* and *nobody.* "I stopped doing my activities for 2 days and now I'm really in pain. I'll never be able to manage my pain." "I feel worse today than I did yesterday. My pain is never going to go away." "I always start a program but then I always quit. Every time is going to be the same, so what's the use?" "Everybody else can do this program. I'm always the one who can't do things." "Nobody can help me."

4. Catastrophizing: When we catastrophize, we react to situations by imagining the worst possible outcome or scenario. "I know that the only option left is to have surgery. I'm sure I'll be laid up for months. Then I'll probably be worse than before." "What if" statements are often catastrophizing in disguise: "What if the operation is a failure?" "What if my pain never gets better, and I have to live like an invalid for the rest of my life?" "What if my spouse leaves me?" "What if I am unable to work?"

5. Control Fallacies: This involves feeling or thinking that one is "externally controlled" by others, such as those in the medical profession, or that one is more in control of the outcomes of problems than one really is. "This new doctor is really going to help me. I know she's the one." "If I don't do it, no one will." "Everyone depends on me. I've got to recover quickly or the family will fall apart."

6. Emotional Reasoning: This line of thinking assumes that what you feel emotionally *must* be true in reality. "I'm taking too long too heal. I must be doing something wrong." "The

pain is back again full force. It's never going to stop." "I'm useless. I'll never be able to
_____ (fill in the blank) again."

7. Filtering: Filtering involves seeing situations through a kind of tunnel vision. Most often,
people filter out any potentially positive aspects of their lives. "This is not living. What's the
use?" (ignoring the sunny day, the phone call from his son, and the delicious breakfast a
neighbor fixed).

8. Entitlement Fallacy: Some level of pain and discomfort is a normal part of life, as are
illness, loss, aging, and eventually death. Some people feel that they are "entitled" to escape
these human experiences (witness the rise in cosmetic surgery). "This kind of pain isn't fair."
"Why do I have to go through this?" "My husband is older than I am and he experiences
relatively no pain. Why am I always the one?"

9. Overgeneralizing: This type of thinking is similar to catastrophizing. Most often, it
consists of assuming that the occurrence of a single event or situation is characteristic of most
if not all others. "I tried twice to use controlled breathing, and I don't feel any better. It's
never going to work." "If today is bad, tomorrow is going to be worse."

10. Mind reading: This involves making assumptions about the thoughts behind another
person's words or actions. "My family avoids talking to me about my pain. They don't really
care about me." "If she really cared, she'd be here rather than out with her friends for lunch."
Contrary to what most people think, it is often more difficult to accept that others care for
us than to think they don't care at all.

These kinds of thinking errors are related to each other, as you may have inferred. In
fact, if you have a tendency toward one line of thinking, you will probably catch yourself
doing one or two of the others. Do any of these ways of thinking seem to characterize your style?

Most people (even people with no pain) tend to use some form of faulty thinking,
especially when under stress. We are going to ask you to label your thoughts in the activities
at the end of this lesson. As you try to label your own thoughts, don't be surprised if it is
confusing at first. It takes practice to identify your thinking errors. Also, although the 10
categories described are a helpful way of showing the most common kinds of thinking errors,
the boundaries between categories often blur. This is another reason that the activities
suggested may be difficult at first.

We focus a lot on thinking in this book because the ramifications are serious. For example,
faulty thinking often leads to poor sleep. How? When you focus on how bad things are, you
are likely to feel more miserable. Uncertainty, worries, and fear keep you from getting to

sleep and staying asleep. Lack of sleeps tires you out so that you can do less the next day. This inactivity further undermines your self-confidence, causes you to lose your hope, and makes you feel helpless and depressed. Meanwhile, your pain is feeling worse.

If you have consistent difficulty falling asleep and you are following a balanced activity and rest program, monitor your thoughts more carefully, particularly before you go to sleep or wake up in the morning. Most people engage in faulty thinking more often either in the morning or at night. Which time makes you most vulnerable to this kind of thinking?

To summarize our discussion so far, your negative or faulty thoughts about your situation can lead to emotions and more thinking that may not match reality. What you think quickly initiates what you feel. What you feel can then often lead to more faulty thinking and to what you do (or don't do) to help yourself. When you catch yourself in negative or faulty thinking, try to just gently label these thoughts as such and move on to a more realistic thought.

Method 2: Behaving Differently

There is an adage, "If you can't feel a certain way, try *acting* that way for awhile." That is because it is easier to act yourself into feeling differently than feeling yourself into acting differently. This does *not* mean being a fake, as you will see further along in this section.

Consider the following: Have you ever noticed in the past that when you feel that you look good in the mirror, you tend to carry yourself differently, and people respond accordingly? On bad pain days, one of our patients wears only his favorite ties to work. These ties make him feel as if he looks good, even when he doesn't feel so good. When he's in the washroom, seeing the tie in the mirror reminds him to smile. Often, he will be complemented on his tie. But is it the tie or the smile?

Another patient of ours always serves herself lunch on her best china on days she feels the worst. It reminds her of the good things in life. Another patient forces herself to reach out at least once to someone else who is having trouble during her "bad weeks." Oddly enough, feelings often follow behavior, so you have more control over how you feel than you may realize.

Your feelings don't have to determine your mood or your behavior. If you are feeling bad, you can still decide how you will respond to your mood and pain. You can still decide whether you will think and behave in a positive way or whether you will surrender to your feelings and think and behave in a more negative fashion. We're not saying it's easy. However, it is good to always be aware that although you can't control situations (e.g., pain, other people), you do have some choices about how to respond inwardly and outwardly. And having choices is always a good thing!

For example, when you feel sad, you can choose to pull the covers over your head. Or you can choose to unburden your heart, or listen to music you love and allow your tears to flow, or write about it in your journal. If you still feel sad, you can choose to feel bitter or you can choose to act yourself into feeling different.

Afterward, you may find yourself thinking, "My sadness has had enough space to express itself; now I'm going to enjoy myself." "My sadness is still here, but I will take a shower, do a few stretching exercises, and dress in my favorite clothes. "I've listened to some sad music and gotten the tears out. Now I think I'll put some more lively music on." It may well be that as you do these things you notice that you are singing or whistling along with the music and feeling better.

Even after funerals, usually at the wake or visitation, people turn from their grief for a while to recall positive features of and experiences with the deceased. Some groups have gatherings when someone dies to celebrate their lives and to recall fond memories as well as to share their grief and loss. Often people are surprised to find themselves laughing at such times. But they shouldn't feel guilty about it. Life goes on. We can choose to live in the moment or dwell in the past or future.

With regard to success in this method, when you feel tired and listless and you go swimming, you have had a successful day, whether or not your mood has changed. When you are in pain and call a friend to listen to her concerns, you have had a successful day, even if your mood has not changed. Success is not measured by moods or by pain but by the courage to take steps despite the pain. Always remember that you have choices.

Let's look once more at this idea of "acting yourself into feeling" for a person without chronic pain. A person who lacks self-confidence can be taught to look, walk, and speak like someone with confidence. As a result, she feels more confident. A shy person who speaks softly and indistinctly and avoids the other's gaze is saying, without words, "I am not important. Don't pay any attention to me." She can be taught to speak up, look into the eyes of the person she is speaking with, and smile. As a result, she feels more outgoing.

Life requires us to play many roles. Sometimes people know only one role, so their range is limited. One person only knows how to clown through unpleasant and distressing emotions. Another person knows only how to be a supporting character, never the star of the play; some people are always trying to be the star. Some people only know how to play serious roles. They can never audition for a romantic comedy. In the theatre of life, it is good to have a flexible set of roles to play, so that you are not just looking on. In other words, don't wait until you have a particular emotion to act the part. Experiment with different behaviors until the part seems to come naturally. Try to remember that thinking differently and behavioral change lead to emotional change.

Exhibit 7.3 illustrates this.

Exhibit 7.3. Effects of Feelings and Behaviors

Feeling	Spontaneous reaction	Result	Desired reaction	Result
Sadness	Being still and alone	Depression	Talking, sharing	Insight, humor
Anger	Bottling it up	Aggression, rage	Telling what you think; telling what you feel	Peace, balance
Fatigue	Long breaks; stuck in a rut	Exhaustion	Short breaks; energetic exercise	Condition improved
Pain	Tightness, sadness, worry	Extreme pain	Relaxed behavior; positive outlook; feeling of control	Bearable pain
Shyness, fear	Avoiding contact, fight–flight	Phobia	Confidently speaking; socializing	Confidence

Method 3: A "Must" is Not a Need!

Albert Ellis, a famous psychologist who focused on helping people change their thoughts, had a humorous saying, "Don't musturbate." When you tell yourself that certain things *must*, *should*, or *have to* be done, you cause emotional pressure and bodily tension and distress. If this tension exceeds a certain level or if it lasts too long, it has a "paralyzing" effect. As a result, you may start to feel overwhelmed. Moreover, these "musts" and "shoulds" cause more pain.

Unrealistic expectations of oneself can be a real burden. This is especially true for younger chronic pain patients with families who used to rely on them for income, housekeeping, cooking, yard work, and so on. They feel that they "should" still be productive, even on very bad pain days. Releasing oneself from such unrealistic expectations can bring surprising relief.

For example, one of our patients felt he "should" continue a foreign language course that he was taking for enrichment. The class formerly met in one place, but that semester it was being held at another. He drove around frantically because he could not find the new location. Finally, he saw a cozy little diner and decided (reluctantly) to ask for directions. Once there, the nice waitress and the happy conversations among the patrons convinced him to have a cup of coffee. He began to relax and realize that he was hungry. The aroma of the home-cooked meat loaf convinced him to order dinner. So what if he was late, he thought. Then, halfway through dinner, he decided to skip the class altogether. He felt slightly guilty but then thought, "The heck with that," and began laughing out loud to himself. It was a hobby, not a job! The whole evening was spent relaxing and enjoying the moment. The next semester, he decided to take a foreign cooking course, which he enjoyed thoroughly.

Activities that you feel forced to perform or feel that you have to do are perceived as more difficult than activities that you feel you have chosen voluntarily. This applies generally but is especially apt for activities in which fear plays a role. Let's consider another parent–child example to illustrate this point.

If your child does not want to eat properly, and you repeatedly and continually insist on his eating nutritious food, he will feel a certain amount of pressure. As a result, he may become steadily more resistant and more obstinate with regard to eating healthfully. In effect, you are rewarding negative behavior with attention.

You increase your chances of being successful in your nutritional goals by phrasing your wish as a choice and rewarding positive behavior. For example, you might say, "You are allowed to choose to eat from what's on your plate, and if you eat something healthy you will receive a nice dessert." In this way, you can encourage your child to eat nutritious food. Make it clear that the child does not *have to* eat the nutritious food on his plate but is *allowed* to eat it. If in addition to the french fries he also eats the spinach and chicken, then he will receive dessert that he likes. The positive attention follows the positive behavior. This may take time, but it is time that is not wasted on rewarding unhealthy behavior (such as nagging when your child refuses to eat).

There are a number of well-entrenched prejudices and misconceptions that lead to people putting too much pressure on themselves. These "musts" and "shoulds" undermine self-respect and make life unnecessarily difficult. Consider the following misconceptions:

- ◆ I *must* be appreciated and loved.
- ◆ I *should* do more. Love depends on what I do, not who I am.
- ◆ I *must* be physically fit, youthful looking, and attractive to be accepted.
- ◆ I *must* achieve something important every day.
- ◆ I *should not* pay attention to myself, as this is egotistical.
- ◆ I *should* give in completely to others' requests.
- ◆ I *should* be self-critical in order to improve.
- ◆ I *should* not praise myself because that is conceited.
- ◆ I *must* learn to live with my pain without complaining.
- ◆ I *must* act as if I feel fine at all times.

Are there any of these misconceptions that you believe? Try picking out one and challenging it on a daily basis.

One of our patients, Julie, who was too dependent on the opinion of others, found a button that read, "What you think of me is none of my business." She kept this by her telephone. It helped her begin to "act real" when she was conversing with someone and not worry as much about their opinions of her.

Consider another of our patients, Lorraine. Lorraine had been working with us for 6 months and had returned to work. Here is her story.

Lorraine has recently started working for an attorney after being out of work for several years because of a back injury. Her boss frequently waits until the last minute to give her an assignment. Then, he expects her to work miracles. It is Friday and, once again, Lorraine has been given an assignment before lunch and an unrealistic deadline to meet. The work must be completed by that evening. Lorraine has plans after work, which makes things even worse.

She begins typing away immediately. She skips lunch and does not take breaks so that she will get it all done in time. She feels her back strain from the buildup of pressure and from sitting in a rigid position. She clenches her teeth, trying to ignore her pain and her feelings. She finds herself thinking,

◆ "My boss should have planned ahead better."
◆ "If I ignore the pain, I can get this done."
◆ "I can't afford to go slowly or take a break because my boss might think I can't do the job."

By the end of the day, Lorraine has not only an aching back but also a pounding tension headache and pain in her jaw from gritting her teeth all day. She cancels her plans and arrives home exhausted. She immediately collapses into bed but has trouble sleeping.

On Saturday, Lorraine remembers some of what we have discussed together about coping with stress, and she begins to think about her day in a different light. She comes up with the following thoughts to replace the ones she had the day before:

◆ "Yes, it would have been nice if my boss had planned ahead better, but that didn't happen. My getting upset about that doesn't help me get through my work. I can manage this."
◆ "Next time I'll stretch and relax in short intervals throughout the day, and the pain won't be so bad later."
◆ "Eventually, I'll need to let my boss know that I have a back injury. He won't think less of me. I'm good at what I do and I always get the work done."
◆ "When we get to know each other better, I'll sit down and discuss how we might get the work done at a less hectic pace."

◆ "Since I missed my outing last night, I'll plan a really nice weekend for myself. I'll call a friend after I have a leisurely breakfast."

What was your reaction when you read the first (Friday) and then the alternative (Saturday) set of self-statements? Did you feel a sense of pressure with the first statements and a sense of relief with the second? Also, did you recognize any of the self-care suggestions we have made in the previous lessons?

Method 4: Stopping at the Right Time

If you push yourself too hard and feel you have to go on with an activity or commitment, you may do harm to the progress that you have achieved. It is important to finish an activity while it is still enjoyable and to stop when it is still fun or at least not painful!

This last suggestion implies that it is important that you have some control over pressure when other people are involved. This was an important thing that Lorraine learned with her work assignments.

It applies as well to social situations. When you go somewhere with someone, for example, let them know that there is a chance that you may want to leave earlier than they will. Ask in advance for the other's cooperation in this regard or suggest that you take separate cars. When you arrive at your destination (e.g., theatre, concert, or movie), try to arrange a seat that will enable you to leave easily if you find it necessary to do so. For example, at a theatre, reserve a seat at the end of the row near the exit. You will notice that the feeling that you are in control (i.e., able to leave) is very liberating in itself and thus reduces tension.

When you are doing something "fun" that you are not really enjoying, give yourself permission to stop (remember our patient who was taking the foreign language course). For example, staying at a party where you are not having fun because of your pain is not a useful strategy. For one thing, you may come to associate going to parties with having unbearable pain. Over time, you may find yourself avoiding social gatherings more and more. If, on the other hand, you leave when you are still feeling good, you give your body and mind the message that parties and socializing are fun.

Letting go of unreasonable demands and acting in your own self-interest allows you to feel more in control of your life and more independent of your pain. You are able to determine what is reasonable to do or not do, maintain a reasonable daily and weekly schedule, and take pleasure in all kinds of activities. You'll do these things not because you should but because you want to.

The risk of forcing yourself beyond your limits is greater in situations where you cannot be yourself or where you are not free to do as you wish. If you have a visitor, you might be afraid of appearing inhospitable if you ask the guest to leave. When you are back at work, you want to make a positive impression, and you cannot just walk away. This means that despite the pain, you do your utmost as well and as long as possible, until it really becomes unbearable.

A result of this can be that visiting others or receiving a visit becomes an emotional burden. Working is associated with excessive pain, so you fear and avoid work. (Ah, now you are starting to understand the power and pervasiveness of the laws of learning!)

You need a safe climate. You can only reduce your disability if you have new, different, successful experiences with visits, work, and other stressful or emotionally charged situations. Only success in these situations will remove the pressure and tension and help you build self-confidence. Not working or not having others over for visits (in short, giving in to your pain) does not really eliminate the pain or even reduce it. On the contrary, by giving in to the pain in this way you reduce self-confidence and will likely experience even more pain (see the next lesson for more about pain and self-confidence).

The ABCD Model

The ABCD model can be a useful tool in helping you deal with pain and other stressors in your life. The model was developed by therapist Albert Ellis to help people with problems other than physical pain. However, we have found it to be extremely helpful in work with our patients with chronic pain. This is how it works:

A is the *"activating event,"* or stressor. It can be physical, emotional, social, or environmental. For our purposes, let's make *A* a muscle spasm in your back that keeps you from fulfilling a commitment.

B is your *"belief system."* This consists of your thoughts and attitudes about the stressor. For example, you may think, "Now I can't do what I said I would. My friends will think I'm weak and always unreliable. I can't do anything right anymore."

C stands for the *"consequences"* of the activating event and your belief system. Consequences are often feelings or emotions. For example, as a result of the kind of thinking described above, you feel down or depressed. You might also feel pain as you tense your back muscles.

D is the way out. *D* means *"disputing"* (challenging, questioning) your negative belief system (the negative thinking that goes on after the stressor). This disputing, in turn, affects how you *feel.* For example, you might question whether your friends will really think that you are weak. You would certainly also challenge the statement "I can't do anything anymore."

How to Use the ABCD Model
in Your Own Life

The ABCD model takes practice but yields extremely positive results over time. As you read this section, we suggest that you start using it whenever you catch a thought that is unhelpful. Use the model on paper in your journal or notebook (see Activity 3 at the end of this lesson for a structured approach). Try to increase the number of times you catch such thoughts.

Some find that using the structured format on paper in the beginning is the key to success. So you may want to give that a try.

Whether you use a chart or simply jot down the As, Bs, Cs, and Ds, you will become acquainted with your belief system. Over time you will more automatically and rapidly dispute the negative thinking that affects how you feel and gets in your way of living life. As you become more familiar with using the model, you will be able to use it without writing, simply working out the ABCDs in your mind.

Let's start with an exercise using the structured format. Try not to skip any steps (e.g., don't jump from B to D).

A. First, write down a recent stressor or event that was followed by a pain flare-up. Keep this concise. A few lines are enough. For example, "I twisted in my chair while reaching for the phone and felt my back strain."

If you're having trouble thinking of a stressor, just go over the past 2 or 3 days when you felt pain. The more recent the stressor, the better able you will be to identify all thoughts and feelings.

B. Next, list all thoughts you may have had when your pain-related stressor occurred. For example, "My back is going out again." "I have to take up the slack and answer the phone for the other secretary who's always out sick." "I thought my doctor said this wouldn't happen if I exercised regularly."
C. Third, jot down all feelings you had right after the stressor. A key to identifying feelings (rather than thoughts) is that when describing feelings you don't usually use the word *that*. If you find yourself saying "I felt that I . . ." you are likely describing a thought, not a feeling. For example, "I thought that the other secretary was faking," is not really a feeling. However, it may contain hints to your feelings. For example, it may contain clues to the feeling "I felt victimized." Notice that you don't say, "I felt *that* I was victimized." "*That*" typically doesn't occur in feeling statements.

Other examples of how you might have felt in this situation are, "I felt angry and disappointed. Later I felt a bit hopeless." You do not need a long list of feelings. A few key ones will do. These feelings are the consequences of your thinking.

D. Finally, you will dispute the thoughts you listed in the second step. You question whether "my back is going out again" is really the case. You might think instead, "My back hurts sometimes. Over time it will get better." Instead of, "My doctor said this wouldn't happen," you might think, "My doctor said that these events will happen less frequently if I keep to my pain management program." And finally, you might question whether the other secretary is *always* out sick." You might think instead, "She's out sick a lot. I wonder if she's struggling with some physical or emotional problem."

As a result of disputing your belief, your feelings may change or become less intense. You may feel, for example, just mildly irritated at the other secretary. You may also feel less hopeless or sad.

As a result of having fewer negative feelings, you will likely be able to think of more positive things you can do for yourself. You might think, for example, "I'll do some relaxation exercises in the ladies' room for a little while." "At lunch, I'll go for a short walk and have a chat with one of my coworkers." "I'm going to trust that I will feel better over time." "I'll seek some diversion and I trust that I'll be alright again in a couple of days."

Work with this ABCD process right now until you feel comfortable with it. Pay particular attention to the fact that the activating event does *not* lead to your feelings. It is your thoughts and beliefs that lead to these feelings. These thoughts represent your *interpretation* of an event. If you are having trouble disputing your beliefs, you might list several possible interpretations of an event and ask yourself, "Which interpretation of the event is most useful to me right now?"

As you go through your day, note when you feel stressed or when you are feeling negative. You can ask yourself the following questions: "What events led up to my negative feelings?" "What did I believe or think about the event that may have led me to become upset?" "Are these beliefs or thoughts really true and accurate?" "Are there other more constructive ways to think about what happened?"

One of our patients, Rose, described a recent event that became a stressor. Let's see how she worked with the ABCD model informally. Note that she had been working with the model for a while, so she didn't need to label the ABCDs, but you can see each as the case is discussed. This case also illustrates some of the stress-reduction and relational issues described in the previous lesson. See you if you can identify them as you read the material.

Rose's husband was on a business trip for four days. She had decided to go on an outing with a good friend the day before he was due home. Rose had a really good time, but that night she needed to take out the trash. She carried a garbage sack that was too heavy to the curb and spent a restless night in pain.

When her husband arrived the next morning, instead of greeting him warmly, she began telling him all the negative things that had occurred while he was away. She didn't even think to tell him about the nice time she had had with her friend. Her husband suddenly remembered that he had promised to fix a widow's broken porch light and told her he would be right back. He was gone for over a half hour, and by this time she was fuming.

She decided to take a hot bath to calm down. She put some lavender soap bubbles in the tub. As she relaxed, she isolated the event that led to her pain. Rose realized that she was blaming her husband for everything that went wrong while he was away. She then felt victimized and fearful ("What would happen if he were to go away even longer?"). That kind of thinking, she thought, had led to her complaining so much when he came home.

Then, when her husband left to help the neighbor, Rose had interpreted his behavior as uncaring. She had thought, "He cares more about a neighbor than he does about me." She then had felt angry and abandoned.

Rose felt stuck for a while at this point, but she knew from past experience that eventually she would work things out. So, she enjoyed the smell of the lavender and the feel of the warm water surrounding her. After a few minutes of relaxing, she began to remember the good time she had had with her friend the day before. She thought about how much her friend really liked her and how good that made her feel. Rose remembered how she had complimented her friend on her new hairstyle.

Then Rose thought of her behavior when her husband had returned home. She had done the opposite of complimenting him. This insight led her to think about his leaving for the neighbor's in light of her own behavior. She found herself laughing and saying to herself, "I guess we both like being around women who appreciate us."

When her husband came home, Rose's pain was still there (although it had decreased after the bath). More important, however, her mood had changed and so did her behavior. She asked her husband about his trip. He came over to the sofa and began talking a little hesitantly. She smiled as he was talking, and he relaxed and took her hand. They both laughed at some of the posturing of his colleagues. By the time they had finished talking, Rose noticed that her pain didn't seem as bad.

This lesson contains a wealth of material that can help you not only deal better with your pain but also improve other areas of your life. It is critical, however, that you not just read this material but put it into practice immediately. In the activities we suggest, we focus more on learning to monitor and identify thoughts and on using the ABCD model than on the other methods that we describe in this lesson.

All of the methods are useful. Once you have the ABCD model mastered, you may want to review the other sections in this lesson. They can only add to your progress over time.

Activities That Can Help

Critical Activities

1. Over the next three days try to jot down in your journal or notebook all of the thoughts that occur to you concerning your pain. Note when and where these thoughts occur.

Try to act as an objective observer while writing down your thoughts. In other words, try not to censor or debate your thoughts; simply write down all the thoughts that come to you. Remember that it takes practice to become familiar with your particular brand of thinking. Automatic thinking is lightning fast. The first day you will likely miss some thoughts. But the second and third day you should have quite a list.

Go over your thoughts and try to label them using the list on pages 133–134. Don't be concerned if some don't fall into a specific category. Just leave an underline to go back to some time later.

Then, over the following 3 days, try to catch your thoughts in stressful situations even if these are not directly related to your pain. Do the same labeling process at the end of the 3 days.

This practice will be invaluable as you get to know your patterns of thinking.

2. Take the thoughts that you recorded in the previous activity and choose one category of thoughts that recur (e.g., catastrophizing). You may want to choose the category in which thoughts occur most frequently. Any time one of these kinds of thoughts comes up in the next week, use your journal or notebook to write down statements to dispute these thoughts. After you become adept at disputing one category of thoughts, work on a second category of thoughts.

We have listed a set of thoughts below that our patients have found useful in disputing their automatic thoughts. See if you can use some of them. See if you can add some of your own that will be useful in the future.

- ◆ "I can cope."
- ◆ "It's no one's fault that I am in pain."
- ◆ "Relax, I can manage my pain."
- ◆ "I have managed this situation before and I can manage it again."
- ◆ "Most people act out of their own motivations. It's unlikely they really meant to hurt my feelings."
- ◆ "I am learning new coping skills each day."
- ◆ "The pain comes and goes. I can outlast it."
- ◆ "No one thinks less of me because I have this pain."

My own disputing thoughts:

_____

_____

_____

_____

_____

Optional Activities

3. If you like a more structured approach, you may want to construct a table in your notebook or journal and keep a diary of stressful situations using the ABCD model.

Date and time	A	B	C	D
9/14, 8:35 a.m.	Back pain while driving	"Oh no my back is going out again." "I'll have to pull over and never get to where I'm going." "I'll be laid up now for weeks."	Fear; anxiety; sick to my stomach	"It will be okay. I may have to take a break and be late. I'll take it easy a bit later."
9/15, 10:30 a.m.	Boss yelled at me	"How could I be so stupid?" "He probably wants to fire me." "There goes my next promotion and raise." " He is always expecting the impossible." "I can't stand much more of this!"	Shame; anger; crying; heart racing	"I feel bad that he yelled at me. He's probably having a really bad day. I'll talk to him some other day when we're both less stressed to see how we can make things go more smoothly in the office. Tonight, I'll take a bubble bath and call a friend to plan an outing."

Note. A = activating event (pain or other distressing situation); B = belief systems (thoughts); C = consequences (feelings, behaviors, physical sensations); D = disputation.

4. Questions to consider.

◆ When you can once again be active (e.g., walk, exercise, do chores around the house) and when you are relaxed and friendly despite the pain, how do you explain to people when you have a setback and act and feel differently?

◆ Do you expect and demand too much of yourself on good days or on bad days? How can you change these expectations?

Gaining Self-Confidence

The transition from tenseness, self-responsibility, and worry
to balance, receptivity, and peace
is the most wonderful change a man can make.
The chief wonder about it is that it so often comes about not by doing,
but by simply relaxing and throwing the burden down.
—William James

*I*f you have worked through all (or a good many) of the lessons in this book, you may be feeling better, if not physically then at least emotionally. Your life is different and, although you may not yet be aware of it, the seeds of self-confidence have been planted. Every day you follow the program, it's like caring for your garden. Eventually your self-confidence will become apparent to you, like the first crocus arriving in spring.

Over time, the pain will become less prominent in the foreground of your life. It will be more like background noise that is bothersome but does not stop you from living a satisfying life. You will have grown from being a person coping with pain to a person thriving despite the pain.

This is all because you have

◆ listened to your body and taken the right steps to respond to these signals;
◆ developed and achieved reasonable goals;
◆ paced your activity and rest cycles;
◆ increased the variety of pleasurable experiences in your life;
◆ improved your relationship with others; and
◆ learned to think yourself into feeling better.

Not only are you developing confidence in yourself, you are also developing confidence in others and in the future in general. In this lesson, you will learn how to hone some of these skills to further build your confidence. We'll start with a brief recap by way of questions to consider and then build from there.

A Daily Inventory

What does your body have to tell you today, right now? Only by carefully paying attention to your body moment by moment, hour by hour, and day by day can you really learn what you need to do to manage your pain.

How do you feel right now? Staying aware of your feelings also helps you to learn important connections between actions (or inactions), thoughts, and stressors.

What are your limitations today? It is important to distinguish, on a daily basis, what your body prevents you from doing (what you are physically incapable of doing) and what your thoughts and feelings prevent you from doing. This helps you to make friends with your body rather than attacking it with thoughts such as, "My back is always acting up and hindering me" (i.e., my back is the enemy). It is important to listen to your body, even if what you hear is not positive. But remember that listening to your body and giving in to discomfort are two different things.

Am I beating myself up today? In the beginning, you were always tough on yourself, beating yourself up in your thoughts when you were unable to do all you expected of yourself. If you are feeling down today, you may be beating yourself up. Ask yourself why. You may be giving more than you have to give, and thus feel depleted. Or you may be having thoughts such as, "I'm such a burden to others. I have to ask for help today." You know yourself better now, and you can identify the kinds of thoughts that may be leading you to feel bad about yourself.

If I am having a bad day today, how can I keep my head above water? At some level, even on bad days, you know that you can only work *with* your body, not *against* it. Think of your body as a child. Care for it as if you were taking care of a child. You nurture the child but you do not coddle it. You listen to your child, not only when the child is happy and healthy, but also when the child has pain and is sick, don't you? Do not be afraid of listening to your pain. It doesn't mean the pain will take you over. You are still in charge.

Learning to Love Yourself

You can only grow to love yourself when you accept and respect yourself as you are. Loving yourself is not holding yourself up to some ideal of what you would like to be at any given time. Try to remember that everyone who does his best at any given time has a right to self-acceptance and respect. You are part of this "everyone." When you do your best, even though it is not "ideal," you still need to give you yourself credit. You may view yourself as a patient when you are having a bad day, but what if you viewed yourself first as a person, a person worthy of your own respect and goodwill despite having limitations because of your pain?

Self-acceptance is the important first step in learning to love yourself. The second step is to invest your time and energy in your own well-being before any other priorities. This investment does not mean that you are being selfish. It means that you are being responsible. Only when we are "full" do we have anything left over to give to others. Only when you respect your own needs can you then respect the needs of others.

We discussed acceptance early in this book. Here it is important to elaborate on that topic, because you will have difficulty building confidence and loving yourself unless you fully understand what acceptance entails.

First, acceptance is an ongoing process. It is not a state that can be achieved for good. Acceptance provides a moment-to-moment climate that permits the possibility of change for the better. It is also a longer term process that entails several stages:

1. *Denial of Limitations.* In this early stage, people act as though nothing has happened to them. They act as if there is no real problem. They hide their condition from themselves and from others, presenting themselves as feeling better than they really feel. They may use painkillers or alcohol to continue denying their pain problem.

2. *Rebellion Against and Anger About Limitations and Pain.* In this stage, a person is aware of the pain and the existence of a problem, but they fight this awareness. They may push their bodies as if they were machines. They may frantically call on all kinds of specialists and feel misjudged and misunderstood by everyone. They keep fighting even if it causes them more pain.

3. *Despondency, Depression, and Passivity.* In this stage, a person may view the pain problem as unsolvable. They feel helpless and hopeless and do not see a way out. They may avoid responsibilities or suffer from sleeplessness during the night. They may increasingly turn to alcohol and other drugs. After a restless night, they may just stay in bed and feel hopeless.

4. *Openness to Adapting to New Circumstances and to Learning New Things.* In this stage, the person becomes more open minded. They decide that they have a problem but that there may be solutions. They may buy a book such as this. They may begin to feel more hope, more control over their lives. They begin to feel better about themselves, and a result, they interact with people differently. Instead of seeing setbacks as failures, they see them realistically, as part of the process of living with chronic pain.

5. *Acceptance.* As a result of going through these stages, they gradually come to accept their body, their situation, and their chronic pain. Instead of fighting, they make peace with their bodies and themselves. This acceptance is a process, so some days, hours, or moments they may be more accepting than others.

It is important to realize that people move back and forth between these stages. That is why we emphasize that acceptance is a process. You will find yourself at different stages of this process at different points in time, even when you are following the advice in this book and even when you are taking good care of yourself. What stage do you feel you are in today, at this very moment?

It is also important to emphasize what acceptance is *not*. Acceptance does not mean that you no longer feel pain or that you no longer see the consequences of having chronic pain. You are still aware of limitations. Not every day is a good day. Acceptance is not pushing yourself beyond realistic limits. It is also not doing less than one is able. Acceptance is not just lying in bed either. Acceptance means just that—that you accept the positive and the negative without needing to deny or exaggerate either.

Becoming Your Own Best Friend

Before you can truly garner appropriate support from others, it is crucial to become your own supporter, your own best friend.

Perfectionism is the enemy in becoming your own best friend. You may not think of yourself as a perfectionist, but you may be surprised. Do you criticize yourself silently when you make a mistake. Do you say things to yourself silently such as "that was dumb" or "I should have known better"? Are your sentences littered with words like "should" or "must"? When others do things to help you, do you sometimes feel resentful because they don't do them like you would if you could? These are all tell-tale signs of perfectionism.

Perfectionism is the enemy, because it is not fair to demand more from yourself than you can achieve. We usually learn to become perfectionists early in life. Sometimes we learn to expect perfection in some areas but not in all areas.

In the past you may have heard, "Make sure that you make a good impression." "What would the neighbors think?" Or, you may have belonged to some highly productive organization, where you encountered much more skill in being self-critical than in being self-confident. One of our patients learned to push herself so hard that when she won a red ribbon in sewing, she felt bad because it wasn't a blue ribbon. Another had had a teacher who stood her up in front of the classroom and said, "Mary, always 99% never 100%."

Unconsciously, such experiences become internalized. That is to say, they become part of your own self, and how you think about yourself and others. Without even being aware of it, you may be operating under the belief that "*What others think is more important than my own opinion.*" "*Only the best is good enough.*" You are a unique human being.

◆ Think a moment about your uniqueness. What is unique about you and how you think, feel, and act. If this is difficult, think about some funny quirk, something positive. Or, just think about the size and shape of your eyes or your laugh or lifelines. It is unlikely anyone else has exactly the same shade and shape of eyes, or the exact placement of laugh or lifelines (don't even think of them as wrinkles). Try to improve the way you talk with yourself given your uniqueness. Even limitations can be considered "unique." When you try and don't succeed, how about saying to yourself in a friendly way "That was a fair try. Trying is more important than succeeding. I like and respect myself for trying. I'll probably do better some other time."

◆ Try not to compare yourself with others or with your "former self."

If a person is continually watched, observed, and evaluated, he or she experiences a lot of stress. If you are constantly doing this to yourself, you will cause yourself unnecessary stress. You'll behave more naturally and feel more relaxed when you are not worried about how you measure up to some arbitrary and unachievable standard or when you are not measuring yourself against others.

If you had siblings or cousins, do you remember how it felt to be "compared" in a negative light? It was unlikely that it made you feel good about your uniqueness or that it really motivated you in a healthy way (being "driven" is not being motivated in a healthy way).

Instead of comparing yourself with others or with your own self, find your own way to be proud of yourself. Seeking and finding your own way will give you confidence. See how it feels to proudly say, "I did it my way and it worked."

You Can't Earn Love

Love is a gift freely given and freely received. If you think that you *must* do your very best to be loved, then your thinking is confused. You then try to *earn* love, you do yourself and often others a great injustice. In fact, you are setting yourself up to fail! Your lovability is not determined by what you *do* or by what you *have*. Being lovable is a given, like the color of your eyes. If someone does not love you as you are (assuming that you are respectful of him or her), then one must question whether they are capable of loving you (or anyone else) right now.

Self-love is most important. Self-love is more about who you *are*, what positive qualities you would like to achieve, and the efforts you make to achieve them. Think for a moment: What kind a person do you want to be? What qualities go into being that person? How can you work toward achieving those qualities? Can you love yourself in the process (rather than just when achieving your goals)?

Although the next question may seem a bit unpleasant, it can be useful to ponder. How do you want your family and friends to remember you if you die before them? Try not to get into the thought of proving something to them (or if you do, you may want to ponder this question: What do you want to prove and to whom?).

It's very satisfying to be able to say to yourself, "I don't have to be as good or better than others. I just need to be myself. I can accept myself as I am, with my imperfections and my limitations and also with all my unique characteristics. That is how I want to be thought of and how I would like to be remembered."

Controlling the Things You Can Control

As we discussed earlier in the book, most things in life are not under our control. But it is helpful to take charge of things that you can control. The following statements are helpful in that regard. Try saying one of them to yourself each day, and see how they "fit."

◆ My situation is not responsible for my mood. I can redirect my thoughts and change my mood.
◆ I am not (my appearance, height, intelligence [IQ], income, health, accomplishments). I am me and that is enough.
◆ What others think of me is none of my business. What is more important is how I think and feel about myself.
◆ I am not responsible for other people's moods or their happiness, but I can be a positive influence on both.

The Problem of Pride

When you have chronic pain, you need assistance at times. But often you may feel diminished and dependent when this occurs. Most people are unaware of it, but this is not a problem of dependency, it is a problem of pride. All of us are dependent on others—*all* of us. From the waitress at the coffee shop to the most powerful politicians, all of us rely on others.

If you have difficulty accepting this, think about electricity. Aren't we all dependent on electricity and on the workers who provide it? Aren't we dependent on farmers and fishers and beef and poultry ranches for our food? "Yes but," you may be thinking, "that's a condition that is shared by everyone. I have to ask for help some days in getting the mail."

First, let's look at what makes it unpleasant to you when tasks and responsibilities that used to be yours have to be taken over by others. Does it make you feel as if you are not indispensable or that you can easily be replaced? Do you begin to feel "less than" or worthless?

Society plays a big role in glorifying (false) independence. If you have bought into this, you are likely to feel sad or angry or depressed when you need help. You may start taking these feelings out on others, who seem so independent to you. You might begin telling them that they are not doing tasks properly or the way you would do it. If your friends and family tell you not to worry, that they will take care of something, do you behave even worse? If they seem frustrated at being interrupted, do you feel ashamed or angry?

These are all signs of false pride. This is nothing to be ashamed of, but it is something to work on. For many people, receiving is more difficult than giving. Does this ring a bell for you? Could you consider that when people help you, you are giving them a gift as well? Feeling helpful is a good feeling. Can you work on receiving help graciously and showing appreciation?

If this is too difficult, find a way to help others first. See how you feel when you make a phone call and listen to someone who feels lonely or sad or anxious without needing to get anything in return. See how it feels when you offer a piece of information to someone who can use it, perhaps through a note in the mail.

Then, the next time someone helps you, try to remember the good feeling you had helping someone else. Even if your helper is grumpy, don't assume that helping you is not helping him or her. Be gracious anyway. If your friends and family tend to help too much, you can ask them to involve you as much as possible. Maybe you can't help in the doing of the task, but you can help in the organization and planning. Also, stress to them that it is helpful to you if they would ask for your advice, counsel, and support sometimes. They may have as difficult a time asking for help as you do!

With your family and with your friends, it's important to think through what you really want and need before you ask them to do something for you. Often people think that they want something concrete when they really want some time and attention. Sometimes people think they want attention, when they really want someone to fix a meal. So, take the time to ask yourself what you really want. Then, find the courage (yes, it takes courage to ask for what you really want) to tell them. In a gentle way, tell the people in your life how they can help, how they can play an important role in your life.

If you still have difficulty with asking for help, you may need to rephrase the way you are asking. Here are some ways that patients have found useful in asking for help:

◆ Would you be so kind as . . .
◆ Would you possibly be able to help me . . .
◆ May I please ask you to do something . . .
◆ I would really like . . .
◆ You would do me a great pleasure by . . .
◆ I would be grateful to you for . . .

Try to remember that when one person is unable to help, think of someone else. It is important to have a range of people whom you can call on for assistance. Interdependence does not pertain to just one person. It means having a network of people with whom you can give and receive.

You can be rightfully proud of yourself when you have learned to ask for help graciously, when you have learned to express appreciation for help, and when you have been able to accept "no" for an answer just as graciously. These capabilities will add to your self-confidence and improve relationships with friends and family.

Learning to Stand Up for Yourself

Many people find it hard to stand up for themselves. Lack of self-confidence, feeling unlovable, fear of conflicts, and a lifetime of habitually not asserting oneself are all obstacles to this important capability.

People who don't stand up for themselves tend to avoid conflicts. They may say *"yes"* when they mean *"no."* They may not agree with something, but for the sake of peace, they give in. However, in the long run they are not able to hide their true feelings. Then, when hurt feelings and frustrations eventually become too much to contain, they are likely to be expressed in the form of an outburst of anger.

The people around them are frightened, and they themselves may be frightened too. They may feel bewildered and embarrassed. They may think, "This is not like me. I don't like that person who just came out. I must never do that again."

When people with chronic pain are not assertive, the people around them start to treat them differently, more as a patient than as a person. People no longer say what they think, but what they think the patient wants to hear. Everyone tries to mind-read, which never works. So, family and friends may avoid the person with chronic pain. Everyone eventually begins to wear a mask that is not natural and is exhausting for everyone.

If this description seems to fit your situation, you may begin to feel that you are not an equal partner in the relationship. Others may feel you are no longer their support and refuge. To begin to change this, it is important to learn how to express yourself and to make your own position clear in each situation that requires this.

When something bothers you or when people are pressuring you to do or say or feel something that you don't, it takes courage not cave in. But, if you want to have a *real* relationship with the people around you and if you want to feel better about yourself, you must begin to say "no." You must begin to challenge people when they behave in ways that are not helpful. Let's focus on saying "no."

In the beginning, this will be hard. You may be awkward. People who are not used to asserting themselves, often say "no" more harshly than they intend when they first try out the word. Think of ways you can say no in a respectful but clear way by reviewing situations in the past when you said "yes" when you really meant "no." How might you have responded differently?

In the beginning, you may want to start with the easiest situations in which to say "no" in your own way. Gradually work up to the more difficult situations. As you do this, you will gain confidence in yourself and feel more in control of the things that are under your control (i.e., your decisions about where to go and what to do).

Balance, Balance, Balance

In all of these situations, it is important to seek balance. For example, in asking for help, try not to move from one extreme (e.g., doing it all by yourself) to the other extreme (e.g., asking others do everything). You can ask people to do certain tasks for you temporarily until you can improve your functioning. You can begin to do small things for yourself that you used to ask others to do for you. And, remember, some days, no matter how well you have followed this pain management program, you may need more help than other days.

Don't start saying "no" to everything when you never said "no" to anything before. Don't try to be assertive with everyone at first. Take your time. Skills and capabilities need time to acquire.

Learning to Problem Solve

Many people assume that "self-esteem" is a feeling. Actually, it is a result of acting in certain ways: nurturing yourself, communicating well with others, being assertive, following through on commitments (especially to yourself), and effectively solving problems, to name a few.

Here we will focus on problem solving. Problem solving is not a natural ability. It is learned. The first step in learning is to begin thinking of problems and conflicts in a different way. If you always see things from the other's point of view, try thinking of the problem or conflict from a different point of view (e.g., an objective observer of the situation). If you always see things from your own point of view, try mentally walking in the shoes of the other person involved in the conflict or problem. Most problems with family and friends are communication problems. It's amazing to learn how often we misinterpret other people and they misinterpret us. One of our patients found it helpful to write about such problems in letters (unsent) between herself and the other person. First she wrote about what happened (the specific behaviors, not the interpretation of the behaviors) and how she felt (not thought) about these. Then, she did the same from the point of view of the other person (again, writing about her behaviors and how the other person may have felt). Next, she visualized the benefits of having addressed the problem or conflict constructively. This three-part exercise

Exhibit 8.1.   The Steps of Problem Solving

Step	Question/Action
1. Problem identification	What is the real problem or concern?
2. Goal selection	How do I feel? What do I want?
3. Generation of alternatives	What can I do? What else can I do?
4. Decision making	Which alternative seems best?
5. Implementation	How can I do this? Do it!
6. Evaluation	Did it work (solve the problem)? If not, what went wrong? Return to steps 1–5.

helped her stay open-minded and kept her from "dumping" her feelings on the other person when it was not the right time to discuss the problem or conflict. These and other problems can benefit from a more structured approach to problem solving as well. Exhibit 8.1 provides a list of stages and questions that are helpful to consider in solving any problem, particularly when you write your answers in your notebook or journal.

Solving the Problem of Pain-Associated Distress

Let's look at this structured method with regard to pain-associated distress. First, redefine the problem (not the pain itself but some feeling, thought, or behavior) as something that is affected by the pain. For example, you might redefine the problem as a conflict with your partner over scheduling or distress about a lack of social activities in your life. Define this problem in specific terms.

For example, in the case of a conflict with a partner, the problem is not "getting along with my partner" but "adjusting our schedules to meet his or her needs and any limitations that I have."

Next, define what you feel and what you want in specific terms as well. For example, in the case of lack of social activities, you might write, "I feel lonely and not part of life. I want to have more people and activities in my life."

Then, generate some ways of solving the problem. Brainstorm a list of at least three ways you might help solve your problem, and don't edit your solutions before you even consider them. Some of our patients have found it helpful to imagine how others in similar circumstances might respond if asked to deal with a similar problem.

From your list, for each proposed solution, evaluate the advantages and disadvantages from your point of view (and, in the case of a conflict with a person, from the point of view of that person as well). Rank the solutions in the order in which you think they might be most likely to solve the problem.

Consider how you might go about putting this solution into practice. Again, it might be good to brainstorm a list. Think through how you might engage in activities to lead to a good outcome, one that resolves the problem.

Then, try out what you believe would be the best and most realistic approach to solving the problem.

Finally, evaluate what happened. Was it successful? Partially successful? Did it fail? If it wasn't fully successful, what might you have done differently? Do you think that one of the other alternatives you generated might have worked better? Why?

If the problem continues to bother you, return to steps 1–5. (For example, you may need to redefine the problem. You might add new approaches to your original list of problem solving alternatives.)

In any case, remember to give yourself credit for making the effort to solve the problem in a constructive way. For example, you might say to yourself, "I've made a good start. I'm not going to sit back and hope or wish the problem would go away. I'll reward myself for trying and then go back to think through the problem again."

Learning From Others

You can learn a lot from people who have already attained success (not perfection) in their lives. The approach these individuals take has been studied, and what has been found is that they possess certain characteristics. These are described here:

Autonomy

Autonomy requires learning to set your own goals. You can involve others, but the final responsibility for your goals and your choices is yours. It also involves letting go of meeting others' expectations of you and being less sensitive to what others think of you. This may be harder than it at first appears, but it is an attribute worth working toward.

Appropriate Risk Taking

This involves being prepared to take risks. People with this characteristic focus more on what they have to gain rather than what they have to lose. Reynolds Price, author of many books of fiction but also an account of his own serious illness (i.e., *A Whole New Life*) learned to take this approach when he became ill. Like other successful people who exemplify this characteristic, Price did not take unreasonable risks, but he did learn to know himself, to be realistic, to weigh outcomes, and to make choices on the basis of these factors.

Realism

Successful people are realistic without being drawn into pessimistic or overly optimistic thinking. They don't aim too high or too low. They pick themselves up when they fail, and they evaluate what they might do better next time. They don't expect to run the marathon unless they have trained systematically.

Present Orientation

Successful people do not dwell in the past, which they consider "history." They are continually active in making realistic plans for the future and who they want to become eventually. They take initiative in making these plans become reality by experimenting in the present.

Focus on Possibilities

Successful people focus on possibilities. Instead of rehearsing the problem over and over, they are most involved in thinking about solutions. They develop talents that enable them to meet challenges, and this makes life seem like a challenge that is interesting and exciting.

Strive for Success

Successful people have the courage to strive for success, even when they encounter major obstacles, such as pain or serious illness. They realize that hope is not enough. They don't have to use hope to goad them into action. Instead of focusing on fear of failure, they focus on discipline and life skills. Mistakes are seen as learning opportunities, rather than reasons to despair.

Summary

You can only learn to live with pain if you regain confidence—confidence in yourself, in others, and in the future. This lesson has reviewed some of the earlier lessons and outlined a number of other ways to regain self-confidence. Read the lesson again when you are feeling down or a bit hopeless. Each time you read it, you may take in a little more.

Activities That Can Help

Critical Activities

1. List two problems that you have been struggling with recently.

(1) _____

(2) _____

Now, use the steps in problem solving described on pages 157–158 and in Exhibit 8.1 to work on these. Write out the steps and your responses in your journal or notebook.

Put your solution into practice and evaluate what went right and what went wrong. Make sure you reward yourself for trying, even if the outcome is less than you hoped it would be

2. Think of a conflict or a problem that you have recently had that involved someone else. Use the same problem-solving steps that you did in the previous activity and record your work in your journal or notebook.

3. If you are unassertive, reread the section on assertiveness. Try saying no to a person you feel safe with. Then, as your confidence in this capability grows, begin saying no to people who tend to intimidate you.

Optional Activities

4. Consider the following question: Today, in which stage of acceptance do you find yourself?

a) denying that there is something wrong
b) rebelling
c) feeling despondent or depressed
d) feeling ready to try new solutions to your problems
e) accepting your situation and yourself just as you are

Putting It All Together

Be not afraid of life.
Believe that life is worth living
and your belief will create that fact.
—William James

*B*efore you started this book, you may have assumed that your pain was solely the result of some physical damage in your body. We have tried to emphasize that physical factors definitely are involved. However, as you have seen as the lessons progressed, there are other elements that contribute both to your pain and the effect that of pain on your physical and emotional functioning.

In this lesson, we bring together all the new insights and behaviors we have shared throughout the book, and we add a few more, such as the effect of the past on the present, problems with motivation, and the finer points of setting goals. Because knowledge is power, we want you to have as much power as you can with regard to your pain and your life. We also are going to stress the importance of humor and taking things less seriously. As the cartoon character Pogo said, "Don't take life too seriously . . . it ain't nohow permanent."

Nonetheless, we will start this lesson on a serious note. Awareness of what we are going to discuss will pave the way for a more joyful and less serious approach to life.

Pain: Past, Present, and Future

Previous pain experiences can influence your current experience of pain and the thoughts and feelings that are associated with that pain. If you ever had to leave a job under adverse conditions (e.g., a layoff, being fired), you probably will never forget the emotions that you experienced. Even after several years in a new workplace, if problems arise you are likely to experience, consciously or unconsciously, a level of anxious arousal. It is as if stressful memories predispose us to experience anxiety in situations that are similar later on. If you have had surgery or if you have had some gruesome experiences with regard to pain (including perhaps some insensitive health care providers), some mental (as well as possibly physical) symptoms are likely still there. These serve as reminders of the distress you experienced. In other words, when you experience pain in the present, you are likely to also experience the effects of memories from previous pain experiences.

However, memory and pain cause distortions. If your pain is very severe now, you may recall your previous pain being less severe. If the pain you feel now is mild, you may recall that the pain you used to experience was worse. Your present pain becomes the anchor by which you judge what your pain used to be like and what you anticipate it will be like in the future. These perceptions feel as if they are true, regardless of objective reality.

Your present pain can also influence what you anticipate (What if this pain gets even worse?) and consequently cause you to limit your activities to prevent pain in the future. However, as we have seen, anxiety and worry open the pain gate, so these anticipations are important to work with (e.g., as described in lesson 7).

It may also be the case that your feelings of pain are telling you something about the present—the here and now. Your body does not protest without reason. Maybe there is too little harmony, security, and balance in your life. It could be that the relationship between your coping resources and ability (what you are able to bear) and your burden (what you have to bear) is out of balance. Numerous other factors in the present can cause your pain to increase—family problems, emotional upset, worry, lack of understanding from your significant others, financial or work problems, or inappropriate activities, to name only a few we have previously described. The pain in the present is telling you to take stock and to shore up your resources (including your coping capabilities).

Even experiences from the past that are unrelated to pain can influence your reaction to pain. The laws of learning we discussed do not just apply to physical pain. The laws of learning help shape our character (i.e., our habitual ways of being and behaving). Are we flexible or rigid? Are we comfortable with some emotions (e.g., sadness) but not others (e.g., anger)? Do we resemble our parents, family members, or other strong authority figures in our ways of dealing with emotions?

We are aware of and can remember only a small proportion of these previous learning experiences. It is the especially negative or distressing experiences that we push out of our conscious memory. This is a matter of survival. Most of us cannot be consciously aware of all the sadness, loneliness, fear, and pain that we have experienced in our lives. Nevertheless, a negative atmosphere growing up, traumatic experiences, and poor coping models do leave their mark. The more intense the experience, the more pain in the family, the greater the influence.

Feelings, as an adult, that you are not allowed to be weak, sick, or afraid of being dependent can be a result of experiences you had growing up. For example, if as a child you had to carry a lot of responsibility in order to survive, then you may find it difficult later as an adult to let go of control with confidence. How might this work in your present life?

Let's say you did have to carry too much responsibility as a child. Now, you may have difficulty asking for help. After you have hurt yourself doing something you weren't ready to do, you might also find yourself saying, "Why am I so stupid? Why did I have to do it all on my own? I should have asked for help." If you were consciously aware in the present of all that had happened to you in the past, you would know that your pattern of independence is understandable. There was likely a period of time when you had to do it all by yourself. You had to do this to survive and function. In other words, in the past there were circumstances in which that independent streak was very appropriate, but now it may be causing you difficulty.

You Have More Power as an Adult

The good news is that as a more consciously aware adult you have more power to create a safe, enjoyable environment in which you can learn more adaptive skills. Some people assume that "you can't teach an old dog new tricks." Some "experts" even proclaim that our character is formed by 3 years of age. But studies have shown that people can change throughout life. People can change in their 90s!

Think about how your pain may have influenced your personality. Likely, it began when you were an adult. Many people we have treated have told us, "I am not the same person I was prior to the start of my pain." Well, positive changes can happen as a result of pain as well.

You may know people who claim they can't change. It is true that people differ in their degrees of ability to change. Each person has different learning histories that shape who they are. The "hardware" (the brain) is roughly the same for most people. But the "software" (past experiences; thinking, feeling, and behavior patterns) is uniquely different for each one of us.

Initially you were "programmed" by your genes, family, and community environment. As you grew up, you began to develop your own preferences; goals; and styles of thinking, feeling, and behaving. The initial software programs, although never entirely erased, can be modified with life experiences.

Many people hate particular programs or patterns they see in themselves or in others. Alcoholics, chain smokers, drug addicts, and pain *patients* (in contrast to people who have pain) may intensely dislike many aspects of themselves or their current lives, but they feel helpless to change. They have yet to take responsibility for their own lives.

As the author James Allen stated,

Each is the architect of his own personality. Not the circumstances, not the problems, not the pain, but the way in which we deal with it, determines our sense of happiness. Happiness is not the absence of pain and cares.

Taking Charge of Your Patterns

Before you experienced chronic pain, you were used to functioning in a particular way. After the pain, you became used to functioning in a different way. Both lifestyles were a set of habits, a part of who you were or are. Most people are attached to their habits, even if they are not good habits. And, as we said, habits are sometimes formed during particular periods of your life and may be difficult to let go of when you reach another period

For example, in young adulthood, it may be necessary and even desirable for people to work really hard. When they retire, unless they have prepared for this transition, they can have a most difficult time and can cause difficulties for those around them.

Pain can have similar results, and that is why we have stressed changing your thoughts, feelings, and behaviors, even if this takes you out of your habitual "comfort zone." If you do not adapt constructively, you can make life harder for yourself and for those around you.

Even good habits can become destructive when followed too rigidly. For example, we have stressed that it is a good idea to spread your work in or outside of the home, your chores, your physical activities, and your errands over the week rather than trying to accomplish them all in one day. Organizing your activities in this way offers important advantages. You accomplish just as much (if not more) but with less strain.

However, if this good habit becomes the driver and you the passenger, even a paced schedule can become a problem. For example, if you have found it helpful to tidy the kitchen thoroughly on a Saturday (rather than trying to clean the whole house that day), and you have a bad day on Saturday, you may feel that you have to tidy the kitchen anyway. You may have decided this not because it is necessary, but because it is Saturday. Your habit, rather than your real need, has become the driver in your life. Flexibility must be a part of a well-balanced life.

If you want to change *bad* habits, a few strategies can be helpful. Ask yourself what this habit helps maintain (fear, pride, perfectionism?). If these feelings are difficult to work through, you might find it helpful to see a counselor for a few sessions. However, what is not helpful with a difficult habit is simply to excuse it by saying "That's just the way I am." That excuse will give you a temporary out, but in the long run it will defeat you.

What is most helpful is to prioritize the habits you want to change and choose one habit to change at a time using the methods we have outlined in this book. The following discussion will be helpful in using all the methods we have discussed.

Motivation 201

Earlier in the book we described why and how to get motivated to make changes. Let's call that *Motivation 101*. This is the next level in learning about that topic—*Motivation 201*.

Let's review first. The amount of effort that you are willing to put in to reach any goal is your motivation. The strength of your motivation is determined by the following:

◆ The clarity of your goal: Exactly what do you want?
◆ The attractiveness of your goal: What are the benefits to you?
◆ The perceived and actual feasibility of your goal: Is it possible or is it realistic, given your current limitations?
◆ Your skill level: Do you have the knowledge and skills necessary to achieve your goal?
◆ Your willingness to persevere: Do you have the courage to continue despite occasional setbacks?

Many people with chronic pain say, "I would do anything to get rid of the pain." But they actually lack what they need to change. Often, they may lack motivation. If you are having difficult putting the lessons in this book into practice, you might review the list above to see if motivation is a problem for you.

The Seasons Change, and So Do You

Try to keep in mind that what you find enjoyable today, this week, or this month may not always be enjoyable. The things that bring us joy are not constants. Sometimes, social contacts bring us joy; other times, solitary pursuits (e.g., hobbies, prayer, meditation) bring us greater joy. Some people use enjoyable activities to motivate themselves to do things that aren't enjoyable (e.g., phoning a friend after they have taken a walk that they didn't look forward to). But after a while, they find that the prospect of the phone call no longer helps them over the hurdle of walking when they don't "feel like" walking. Then, it is time to think of new ways of bringing oneself joy. If your joy recipes are limited, then you have less with which to spice up your life. That is why it is helpful to sample regularly from the menu of life's small joys.

Other ways of staying motivated include becoming more knowledgeable over time. We have stressed throughout this book the importance of both others' knowledge about pain and your own personal knowledge of pain. It helps to update your knowledge bank from reputable sources when you are feeling bored with your pain management program.

But it is also helpful to gain knowledge in any area in order to keep your mind sharp and your interests lively. It is best to do this when you are not in a down period or having a bad day. It's hard to motivate oneself to learn a new skill or body of knowledge when things are going poorly.

Instead, when things are going well or you are having a good day, begin to think about what you would like to learn to do or what you would like to study. Some television can be relaxing, but a daily overdose of television can be deadly to mind and spirit.

Perhaps you have always been interested in the history of quilting, but have never found the time to explore this. Perhaps your interests are in archaeology. Don't feel you have to have training or a college education to explore your interests. Just begin where you are and build knowledge and skills that will later serve as resources when other areas of your life are not so good.

What does this have to do with pain? When pain is unavoidable, distraction can be one's most useful ally. However, you must become acquainted with your ally when you are not in pain in order to feel comfortable turning to your ally when distraction is truly needed.

Motivational problems sometimes stem from not knowing how to set goals. Although we cover the basics of this topic in lesson 2, there are some finer points that you may want to consider.

The Mechanics of Goal Setting

Remember that most people need both short-term and long-term goals to feel successful. It is helpful to formulate your goals in terms of daily, weekly, monthly, biannual, and annual goals.

It is also critical that you formulate your goals in terms of effort, not in terms of results. This is because we have control over our efforts, but we do not have complete control over the results (although some patterns of effort are more associated with success than others, e.g., pacing).

Place your goals, especially your daily, weekly, and monthly goals, in a prominent place, so you are reminded on a daily basis of what you are trying to do. Periodically review your monthly and annual goals to remind yourself of what you are working toward.

Making copies of the activity, relaxation, and progress charts provided early in this book are useful tools to keep track of progress toward goals. These, too, can be posted in prominent places, and a notebook containing tabs for each month can help you keep track of progress in your thinking and behavior.

Most people find that it helps to have an attractive or personally meaningful cover for their journal or their notebook in which they keep their goals and progress charts, so that they are apt to keep it out to review regularly. A three-ring binder that allows you to insert a picture or some other item on the front cover allows for changes over time. These can be found in most office supply stores.

As you see progress in moving closer to achieving your goals, your motivation will increase. When you see connections between helpful patterns and positive benefits, your motivation will increase as well. The sense of accomplishment (i.e., consistent efforts) will help build self-esteem.

Our patients have taught us that goals work like magnets. The closer they get to them, the stronger the attraction.

Summary

Pain is an important messenger, and pain management is the critical skill you need to decode your pain's message and thrive despite the pain. That, in a nutshell, is what this book is all about.

Some of you may have read this book without doing any of the activities. That's okay for now. Your timing may be off with regard to change, and you may need to come back to this book at a later time when you are more ready. But keep this book in a safe place. We are here to work with you when you feel able to do so.

Others of you may have been working through the book consistently. You have likely seen changes in your thoughts, feelings, and behaviors first and in your experience of pain next. For these readers, we offer a last lesson on maintaining the positive changes that have been achieved by following the lessons in this program.

As most dieters know, the initial pounds are easier to lose than the later ones. And keeping weight off for good is more difficult than losing it in the first place. So, please don't skip the next lesson. It's just as important as the rest.

Activities That Can Help

Critical Activities

1. Think about a habit of yours that has been difficult to change. Then, list some of the ways to motivate yourself that we describe in this lesson. Pick one or two and try them for at least 6 weeks (it takes at least 6 weeks to change an ingrained habit). At the end of that time, record in your notebook or journal how and why you were successful in changing.

2. If you are one of the readers who has not tried any of the activities so far, consider why this is so. Are you going through a very demanding time but will do the activities as soon as you can catch your breath? Do you tend to put yourself last on your list of priorities and perhaps need to rethink that? Do you tend to procrastinate and need to work on that? Or are you one of those people we found depicted in a cartoon once: Given the choice of entering the door marked "heaven" and entering the door marked "reading about heaven," do you tend to choose the latter? If so, have a laugh at yourself and turn to the activities at the beginning of lesson 1.

3. If you have discovered particular problems with regard to your past that may be contributing to your difficulty in practicing this program, write about these in your journal or notebook. If you are still having problems, consider short-term counseling with a therapist familiar with pain management as well as with general problems of the past influencing the present.

Optional Activities

4. Choose one or two of the suggested readings or audio programs listed at the end of this book. Check them out from the library or order them from your local bookstore or on the Internet.

The Importance of Maintenance and "Setbacks"

Change is a process, not a discrete event.

Success in managing pain is dependent on an individual's capacity to adjust and to make changes as needed. For chronic pain, we have seen that changes may be necessary in just about every area of life—your daily activity and rest habits, the way you choose to think about your pain, and the way you relate to others, to name only a few.

In this lesson, we stress *maintenance*, which is the last step in the pain management program. We review the three most important pain management principles. We also discuss how periodic relapses are in some sense normal, although we help you to experience as few setbacks and relapses as possible.

The Top Three Pain Management Principles

Principle 1: Bringing More Physical Activity or Exercise Into Your Life

Pain reduction comes about when you are reasonably able to exert yourself physically despite some discomfort or pain. Exercising within your limits can be therapeutic both physically and mentally. The keys to success in this regard are being active *regularly* and *consistently*. Our patients have taught us that if they establish a schedule and stick with it, they invariably feel pain less often and less intensely.

Principle 2: Ensuring Sufficient Relaxation

Pain reduction occurs when you are able to relax despite the pain. Acceptance and peace can't coexist with struggle and tension. Our patients have taught us that balancing activity and rest and finding time each day for relaxation and enjoyment are crucial to pain management.

Principle 3: Bringing More Diversion and Fun Into Life

Pain needs competition—diversions that help you focus on the things that are going well in your life or that create opportunities for well-being mentally and emotionally. This changes the scene from pain in the foreground and life in the background to life in the forefront and pain to the rear. Our patients have taught us that boredom and being stuck in a rut are roadblocks to successful pain management. Most people find the first two principles the easier ones (note we do not say "easy") to implement. The third principle gives many people the most problems. Consider the case of Fred.

> Fred had significant pain problems when his wife suddenly died. He was barely able to provide essential care for his three children. One evening, his son approached him about helping with a school project. Fred rudely sent him away—he was preoccupied with his pain and his loss. However, his son kept on badgering him. Troubled by vague guilt feelings about not paying attention to his children, Fred decided to try to get involved in the school project. He soon found that it was more complicated than he would have thought. He decided to break the project into manageable segments. Fred worked on the project with his son for half an hour before his son had to go to bed. Fred promised that he would continue to work on the project. It took him until two o'clock in the morning. Fred felt a sense of satisfaction. He crept upstairs and proudly placed the finished project next to his son's bed. While working on the school project, Fred did not focus on his pain. The pain did not disappear, but it faded into the background. It was no longer the focus of his attention.

You need the healthy tension that is realized by social contact, creativity, and, yes, fun. Fun, as Fred learned, can be as unpredictable as the weather. One just has to decide to "go outside" of oneself to discover it. Developing hobbies, stimulating creativity, deepening social contacts, playing games, becoming adventuresome, talking, laughing, and even reading and writing can bring fun and color into your life

For each person, what is fun will differ. Some find satisfaction in quiet pursuits, whereas others like the hustle and bustle of being in a crowd. If you are having difficulty with this pain management principle, remember to seek activities that fit you, but don't be afraid to step out of your comfort zone once in a while. Here are some additional pointers:

◆ Are you especially interested in concrete things? Are you practical? Activities such as crafts, car or motor repair, model building, sewing, woodworking, and quilting are practical and creative as well.

◆ Do you enjoy learning new things? Activities such as chess, bridge, crossword puzzles, and Scrabble often appeal to people who like to stretch their minds and learn new things. Other food for the mind can be found in libraries and on the Internet. (Be cautious with the Internet, however. There is also a lot of "junk food" online as well.) Mentally, you can go on voyages of discovery to far away, foreign regions; you can go back in time, to earlier civilizations; you can share the thoughts of the great thinkers; you can bury yourself in countless subjects or specialize. Especially when you are less able to be continuously physically active, enriching your mind can be a powerful antidote to pain.

◆ Do you have artistic interests? Activities such as drawing, painting, music, drama, and literature are examples of artistic interests. You don't have to actually "create" to be creative. You can simply enjoy the creations of others. Being artistic includes "being" as well as doing. If you haven't considered such activities before, try to have an open mind. Try out different areas. There is a saying that is apt here: "The unknown is unloved."

◆ Are you interested in social activities? Volunteer work of all kinds, club membership, community center activities, special interest groups, or classes are examples of "fun" that might appeal to you once you've given them a chance. If you have a talent for organizing, volunteering for service clubs, political parties, community action groups, and the like, there are many opportunities for you to have fun doing what you do best. The main thing is to ensure that you have people in your life and that you keep meeting new people periodically. If getting around town is too difficult, write letters, telephone people, ask them to drop by. People are unlikely to visit unless invited. Take the initiative on your good days; later, even on your bad days you will find social companionship comforting.

◆ Do you like to work with numbers? Activities include starting collections, volunteering to be the treasurer for an interest group, joining or helping set up an investment club, and so forth.

◆ Do you have interests in nature? Are you interested in everything that lives and grows? You might choose to put some effort into container gardening, keeping an aquarium or terrarium, keeping a pet bird or cat (but not both!), putting together a herbarium, fishing, and ecological activities, among others.

In Exhibit 10.1, we include some additional examples of different activities that were suggested by our patients. By no means should these be viewed as a complete list of interests and activities. You may have some ideas that are very enjoyable that we have not even hinted

Exhibit 10.1. Partial List of Pleasurable Activities

Hobbies

Do artwork	Write poetry, plays, short stories
Make pottery or ceramics	Learn and sing songs
Knit or do needlework	Play a musical instrument
Photography	Start a collection of things that interest you
Redecoration	Work in the garden or with houseplants
Cooking	Join a group or organization that shares your interests
Do woodwork or carpentry	
Repair motors, clocks	Visit an art gallery or museum

Entertaining Activities

Watch television	Go to a zoo or aquarium
Listen to the radio, records, tapes, or CDs	Go to a sporting event, races
Go to the movies, a play	Go to a concert or ballet

Social Activities

Spend time with your children, grandchildren, nieces, or nephews	Make dinner or a party for friends
	Join a club
Write, telephone, or e-mail friends	Join a self-help group like the American Chronic Pain Association[1]
Have lunch with a family member or friend	
Visit neighbors or friends	Go to a bar or tavern
Invite neighbors or friends to visit you	Go to a party or on a picnic
Go to church, synagogue, temple, or mosque	Play cards, checkers, or chess

Educational Activities

Read books, plays, poems, magazines, short stories	Take a class in an area that interests you
	Learn a foreign language
Read the Bible, Koran, or religious texts	Look up information on topics that interest you in the library or Internet
Go to a lecture in an area that interests you	

Additional Activities

Take care of a pet	Have your hair done
Go for a drive in the country	Spend time outdoors
Take a trip (short or long)	Rearrange things in your house
Go shopping at a mall or one of your favorite stores	Make food or crafts to give away or sell
	Have a meal in a restaurant
Can, freeze food, or make preserves	Go camping
Buy something for yourself or others	Say prayers

continued

Exhibit 10.1. Partial List of Pleasurable Activities *Continued*

Additional Activities *Continued*

Go people watching at a park or mall

Go to a health club or sauna

Learn to do something new

Talk on the telephone

Watch birds or animals

Play a board game (for example, Monopoly, Scrabble)

Play table tennis

Go swimming

Start a new project

Go to a casino

Listen to the sounds of nature

Have a lively conversation

Walk in the woods, mountains, or by the sea or lake

Go fishing

Go bird watching

Write letters

Take a walk

Go to a garage sale

Do volunteer work

Travel with a group

Teach something to someone

Copy your recipes for others

Go on a nature walk

Other Activities

Now list other activities that come to your mind.

[1]American Chronic Pain Association, P.O. Box 850, Rocklin, CA 95677, http://www.theacpa.org/

at. Many others that we list will be of no interest to you whatsoever. What is important is for you to have a list of enjoyable activities that fit you and from which you can choose on a daily basis.

To sum up, when you can no longer perform what used to be your "normal activities," you will likely have a sense of empty space in your life. If nothing pleasurable is found to replace these activities, negative emotions such as irritability, depression, or sadness may fill up this space. Sometimes it takes a serious jolt to be released from these emotions. Then, unexpected sources of strength and energy are found. The case of Eileen below shows how this happened to one of our patients. We hope that you won't wait for such an event to begin enjoying life and unearthing strengths and talents that you may not even know that you possess!

Eileen took part in our pain management program and was determined to improve her life. However, she was stuck. No matter what she tried, she felt her situation deteriorating. Walks became shorter; she started using crutches and eventually needed a wheelchair.

A few months after starting our program, her son was involved in a serious car accident. During Eileen's difficulties, her son had always been a great support. Now he needed her help. To her own surprise and those who knew her, the new task, the new demands, released unexpected energy.

The "What, How, and When" of Staying Involved in Life

When you have a clear picture of the kinds of activities that interest you, it is important to make a choice and a plan. Ask yourself concrete questions:

- ◆ "What do I want to do?"
- ◆ "How will I accomplish this?"
- ◆ "When will I start?"
- ◆ "What do I need to do to get going?"
- ◆ "What problems might get in my way?"
- ◆ "What can I do about potential problems that I anticipate or that arise unexpectedly?"

It often helps to tell others what you want and plan to do on a daily basis. Seek advice and encouragement from others. Each evening take a look at what pleasurable activities you included in your day. How far did you get with your plans? Do your plans need adjusting? How might you bring even more pleasure into your daily life?

Managing Flare-Ups

Most of our patients do experience periodic episodes of worsening pain, occasional sleeplessness, and morning stiffness. These flare-ups are temporary, and, if managed well, are typically followed by improvement. When flare-ups occur, it is important to take an active approach to managing them. At first, you may feel distressed that pain has returned or gotten worse. You might worry that the pain has returned full force and will never remit. In your darkest moments, you may feel that all is lost—that the skills you learned in this book have been of no use whatsoever. In your brighter moments during flare-ups, you might remember what we said about Murphy's Law: "If something can go wrong it will." And Mrs. Murphy's commentary on Murphy's Law? "Murphy was an optimist!"

But seriously, let's look at causes of flare-ups. Flare-ups are sometimes caused by identifiable aggravating factors. A weekend doing too much yard work or the physical stress of repetitive motion (e.g., too many hours at the computer) may be followed by increased pain and stiffness. Emotional stress, such as conflicts with family or friends, may also exacerbate pain and lead to sleeplessness. Certain weather conditions may set off a flare-up. However, many times flare-ups occur with no identifiable cause. In these cases, it is best not to spend too much time analyzing what caused the flare-up, because this may actually increase the pain.

If you do identify specific factors that clearly aggravate your pain, you can possibly reduce them in the future by avoiding or limiting certain activities, making a plan to deal differently with conflict, and so on.

Before the next flare-up occurs, the most important thing you can do is to develop a personal *flare-up management plan*. In Exhibit 10.2, we describe a typical plan. Note that this is only one example. You are unique, and you need to develop plans specifically for you. It can be helpful to go over your plans with a nurse, doctor, or physical therapist. This kind of planning ahead is called *relapse prevention* in many fields, including pain management.

After a flare-up, it is important to rest and recover (for a reasonable, limited time while still maintaining activity using your pacing skills). It is also important to review what was effective and to commend and comfort yourself for having weathered the increased pain.

Exhibit 10.2. Sample Flare-Up Management Plan

◆ Change activity–rest cycle to decrease activities by one half.
◆ Cut back on physical exercises by a certain amount—check with a physical therapist to determine amount.
◆ Over 3 days, gradually increase activities up to level prior to flare-up.
◆ Practice relaxation and controlled breathing exercises twice as often as before flare-up.
◆ Increase use of other pain coping skills such as distraction, imagery, and positive thoughts.
◆ Increase frequency of relaxing activities.
◆ Inform family that you are having a flare-up and what you will be doing about it.
◆ Tell significant others what they can do to help you during the flare-up.

But what do I do during a flare-up? This is a reasonable question. During a flare-up, relying on your newly developed qualities, such as acceptance, is critical. Remembering that pain and distress are a necessary part of life and that they cannot be entirely avoided can be helpful. Remembering that you are not alone in the world of chronic pain is helpful as well.

Acceptance of pain when you are having extremely high levels of discomfort is never easy. But our patients have taught us that if they try to observe the pain without trying to change it, they feel better than when they are frantically seeking control over the pain. They have told us that it is better to observe their thoughts and feelings than to act on them impulsively. They have told us that acceptance may not decrease pain, but it may decrease suffering.

You may have heard the adage, "Pain is necessary, but suffering is optional." Pain and suffering are not the same thing. Pain is the physical hurt you feel; suffering is when you tell yourself lies about pain (e.g., it will never go away) and judge yourself harshly for having pain. Suffering is when you blame other people who are not to blame or when you try to control people, places, or things that are not under your control. Pain is unavoidable at times. Suffering is a result of the lack of acceptance of that pain and associated feelings and emotions. Suffering also occurs when you forget that there is more to life than even intense pain. Suffering decreases by engaging in pleasurable activities that soothe and satisfy your senses, such as listening to music, stroking a pet, watching a relaxing show on television, burning a candle with an aroma you enjoy, having a cup of your favorite fruit or ice cream, or getting or giving a massage (even a foot massage can be highly pleasurable).

When you find out that you are able to put your flare-up management plan into action, that you are able to bring rest, harmony and also fun back into your life, despite pain, then you know that you are accepting life on life's terms. While you may be in pain, you will not necessarily be suffering! You will identify with the prayer with which we began this book: "Grant me the SERENITY to accept the things I cannot change; COURAGE to change things I can; and WISDOM to know the difference."

A Final Word

Your investment of time and energy in this pain management program and your commitment to your own well-being have made you a different person than you were when we first met you in this book. Regardless of flare-ups, setbacks, and other unexpected challenges, what you have accomplished is IRREVERSIBLE!

We encourage you to return to review the different lessons periodically, because you may find new things each time you reread a lesson. We have shared a tremendous amount of information. We hope to hear from you about what worked and what didn't! Remember, we're all in this together! (And yes, there is homework in this lesson as well. Darn!)

We have listed key points of this self-management program. You might want to copy it and place it someplace where you will see it frequently so that it can serve as a reminder.

Key Points to Remember

◆ Be alert to the erroneous myths about pain.
  * Pain is *not* a reliable signal of injury.
  * The absence of injury or disease does not mean that your pain is not *real—All pain is real.*
  * Your pain should be taken seriously.
  * There is a no pill for every ill, "when in doubt cut it out" is not a useful way to treat chronic pain.
  * Hurt and harm are not equal.
  * If you have had pain for a long time, there is much you can do about it—you are *not* helpless and hopeless.
◆ Know your limits—balance overload and underload to find the optimal load for you.
◆ You are a *person* not a *patient*!
◆ Maintain a regular exercise plan that gradually increases until you reach an optimal level; stay with it; keep charts where you record the amount of your exercise.
◆ Move it or lose it!, but *exercise smarter not harder.*
◆ *Pacing* of activity and energy is important, balance activity and rest (relaxation).
◆ Maintain a regular sleep schedule.
◆ Practice relaxation and controlled breathing exercises on a daily basis.
◆ Increase pleasant activities.
◆ Communicate with significant others—rely on *sharing,* not *mind-reading.*
◆ Be aware of the *Laws of Learning* and the role of *attention, anticipation, and fear.*
◆ Thoughts, feeling, behavior, and the body are related. The *pain gate* can be open or closed by each of them.
◆ Change painful thoughts into realistic ones.
◆ Build up your "wants" and avoid the "Tyranny of Shoulds and Musts."
◆ Accept yourself and your limitations; the new you may be different from the old but not worse.
◆ Reward yourself for your efforts and not just the results.
◆ Expect relapses, setbacks, and bad days, but do not let them defeat you!

Be yourself, act like yourself, and like yourself, so you can take good care of yourself!

Activities That Can Help

1. Make three plans.

    a. A plan to systematically become more active over time (indicate what, when, where, how much, and for how long).

        _____

        _____

    b. A plan to bring even more fun and relaxation into your life (indicate what, when, where, how much, and for how long).

        _____

        _____

    c. A plan to deal with inevitable flare-ups (i.e., your relapse prevention plan). List the options, skills, and techniques you can use. Be as specific as you can. Place this in a prominent location so that you can refer to it immediately when you need to.

2. Schedule a check-up with yourself on your pain and follow through with your appointment.

Record your ratings on the scales that follow.

1. Rate the level of your pain at the **PRESENT MOMENT**.

     0   1   2   3   4   5   6

    No pain   Very intense pain

2. In general, during the **PAST WEEK** how much did your pain interfere with daily activities?

| 0 | 1 | 2 | 3 | 4 | 5 | 6 |

No interference   Extreme interference

3. During the **PAST WEEK**, how much has your pain changed the amount of satisfaction or enjoyment you get from taking part in social and recreational activities?

| 0 | 1 | 2 | 3 | 4 | 5 | 6 |

No change   Extreme change

4. On average, how severe has your pain been during the **PAST WEEK**?

| 0 | 1 | 2 | 3 | 4 | 5 | 6 |

Not severe   Extremely severe

5. During the **PAST WEEK**, how well do you feel that you have been able to deal with your problems?

| 0 | 1 | 2 | 3 | 4 | 5 | 6 |

Not at all   Extremely well

6. During the **PAST WEEK**, how successful were you in coping with stressful situations in your life?

| 0 | 1 | 2 | 3 | 4 | 5 | 6 |

Not successful   Extremely successful

7. During the **PAST WEEK**, how irritable have you been?

| 0 | 1 | 2 | 3 | 4 | 5 | 6 |

Not irritable   Extremely irritable

8. During the **PAST WEEK**, how tense or anxious have you been?

| 0 | 1 | 2 | 3 | 4 | 5 | 6 |

Not anxious/tense   Extremely anxious/tense

Now, go back to your ratings after lessons 1 (p. 27), and 5 (p. 111) and in the space below record the numbers you reported previously for each of the two rating periods in the space below.

1. Rate the level of your pain at the **PRESENT MOMENT**.

        0   1   2   3   4   5   6

     No pain   Very intense pain

After lesson 1   After lesson 5   Now

_____   _____   _____

2. In general, during the **PAST WEEK** how much did your pain interfere with daily activities?

        0   1   2   3   4   5   6

     No interference   Extreme interference

After lesson 1   After lesson 5   Now

_____   _____   _____

3. During the **PAST WEEK**, how much has your pain changed the amount of satisfaction or enjoyment you get from taking part in social and recreational activities?

        0   1   2   3   4   5   6

     No change   Extreme change

After lesson 1   After lesson 5   Now

_____   _____   _____

4. On average, how severe has your pain been during the **PAST WEEK**?

        0   1   2   3   4   5   6

     Not severe   Extremely severe

After lesson 1   After lesson 5   Now

_____   _____   _____

5. During the **PAST WEEK**, how well do you feel that you have been able to deal with your problems?

| 0 | 1 | 2 | 3 | 4 | 5 | 6 |

Not at all   Extremely well

After lesson 1   After lesson 5   Now

____   ____   ____

6. During the **PAST WEEK**, how successful were you in coping with stressful situations in your life?

| 0 | 1 | 2 | 3 | 4 | 5 | 6 |

Not successful   Extremely successful

After lesson 1   After lesson 5   Now

____   ____   ____

7. During the **PAST WEEK**, how irritable have you been?

| 0 | 1 | 2 | 3 | 4 | 5 | 6 |

Not irritable   Extremely irritable

After lesson 1   After lesson 5   Now

____   ____   ____

8. During the **PAST WEEK**, how tense or anxious have you been?

| 0 | 1 | 2 | 3 | 4 | 5 | 6 |

Not anxious/tense   Extremely anxious/tense

After lesson 1   After lesson 5   Now

____   ____   ____

Have these numbers gone down, remained the same, fluctuated, or gone up? If they have gone down great, but if they have fluctuated or gone up it would be worth your effort to try to identify what factors may have affected them. Remember to think about your behavior, thoughts, and feelings during each of the weeks that you recorded your pain and responses.

Additional Reading

Lesson 1: Becoming Your Own Pain Management Expert

Melzack, R., & Wall, P. D. (1982). *The challenge of pain.* New York: Basic Books.

Lesson 2: Activity, Rest, and Pacing

Bliss, E. C. (1978). *Getting things done.* Bantam Books: New York.

Christy, D., & Sarafconn, C. A. (1990). *Pacing yourself: Steps to helping save your energy.* Bloomington, IL: Cheever Publishing.

Inkeles, G., & Schencke, I. (1994). *Ergonomic living: How to create a user-friendly home and office.* New York: Simon and Schuster.

Hage, M. (1992). *The back pain book.* Atlanta, GA: Peachtree Publishers.

Lycholat, T. (1995). *The complete book of stretching,* Ramsbury Marlborough, England: Crowood.

Oliver, J. (1994). *Back-care: An illustrated guide.* Boston: Butterworth-Heinenman.

Ornstein, R., & Sobel, D. (1989). *Healthy pleasures.* Reading, MA: Addison-Wesley.

Reynolds, D. K. (2002). *A handbook for constructive living.* Honolulu: University of Hawaii Press.

Rippe, J., & Ann Ward, A. (1989). *Rockport's complete book of fitness and walking.* New York: Prentice-Hall.

Ryan, M. J. (2003). *The power of patience.* New York: Random House.

Schaef, A. W. (1990). *Meditations for women who do too much.* San Francisco: Harper.

Wilson, A. (1994). *Are you sitting comfortably? A self-help guide for sufferers of back pain, neck strain, headaches, RSI, and other health problems.* London: Optima.

Lesson 3: Learning to Relax

Achtenberg, J., Dossey, B., & Kolkneier, L. (1994). *Rituals of healing. Using imagery for health and wellness.* New York: Bantam Books.

Benson, H. (1976). *The relaxation response.* New York: William Morrow.

Casey, K. (2001). *Each day a new beginning: A meditation book and journal for self-reflection.* Center City, MN: Hazelden.

Davis, M., Eshelman, E., & McKay, M. (1995). *The relaxation and stress reduction workbook* (4th ed.). Oakland, CA: New Harbinger.

Fanning, P. (1994). *Visualization for change* (2nd ed.). Oakland, CA: New Harbinger.

Gates, R., & Kenison, K. (2002). *Meditations from the mat: Daily reflections on the path of yoga.* New York: Random House.

Kabat-Zinn, J. (1990). *Full catastrophe living.* New York, Delta Books.

Ruhnke, A., & Wurzburger, A. (1995). *Body wisdom: Simple massage and relaxation techniques for busy people.* Boston: Charles Tuttle.

Weintraub, A. (2004). *Yoga for depression: A compassionate guide to relieve suffering through yoga.* New York: Random House.

Young, S. (1995). *Break through pain: How to relieve pain using powerful meditation techniques* [Audio-tape]. Louisville, CO: Sounds True.

Young, S. (2004). *Pain relief* [Audio CD]. Louisville, CO: Sounds True.

Lesson 4: Are You Always Tired? Ways to Combat Fatigue

Baird, P. (1993). *The pyramid cookbook: Pleasures of the food guide pyramid.* New York: Henry Holt.

Catalano, E. M., et al. (1990). *Getting to sleep.* Oakland, CA: New Harbinger.

Hauri, P., & Linde, S. (1991). *No more sleepless nights.* New York: Wiley.

Jacobs, G. (1998). *Say goodnight to insomnia: The six-week, drug-free program developed at Harvard medical school.* New York: Holt.

Lamberg, L., & the American Medical Association. (1984). *Straight-talk, no-nonsense guide to better sleep.* New York: Random House.

Regestein, Q., Ritchie, D., & the editors of Consumer Reports Books. (1990). *Sleep: Problems & solutions.* Mount Vernon, NY: Consumer Union.

Somer, E. (1996). *Food & mood: The complete guide to eating well and feeling your best.* New York: Holt.

Lesson 5: Don't Let Pain Ruin Your Relationships!

Bower, S. A., & Bower, G. H. (2004). *Asserting yourself.* Reading, MA: Addison-Wesley.

Hendrix, H., & Hunt, H. L. (2004). *Receiving love: Transform your relationship by letting yourself be loved.* New York: Atria Books.

Lange, A., & Jakubowski, P. (1976). *Responsible assertive behavior.* Champaign, IL: Research Press.

Lerner, H. (2001). *The dance of connection.* New York: HarperCollins.

McKay, M., Davis, M., & Fanning, P. (1995). *Messages: The communication skills book* (2nd ed.). Oakland, CA: New Harbinger.

Pennebaker, J. (1990). *Opening up: The healing power of confiding in others.* New York: William Morrow.

Tannen, D. (1986). *That's not what I meant!: How conversational style makes or breaks relationships.* New York: Ballentine Books.

Tannen, D. (1990). *You just don't understand: Women and men in conversation.* New York: William Morrow.

Williams, R., & Williams, V. (1993). *Anger kills: Seventeen strategies for controlling the hostility that can harm your heart.* New York: Times Books.

Lesson 6: Changing Behavior

Armstrong, L., & Jenkins, S. (2000). *It's not about the bike.* New York: Berkley.

Bridges, W. (2003). *Managing transitions: Making the most of change.* Cambridge, MA: Perseus.

Ilardo, J., & Rothman, C. (2003). *Take a chance: Risks to grow by.* New York: MJF Books.

McKay, M., Davis, M., & Fanning, P. (1981). *Thoughts and feelings.* Richmond, CA: New Harbinger.

Nicholas, M., Molloy, A., Tonkin, L., & Beeston, L. (2000). Manage your pain. Sydney, Australia: ABC Books.

Price, R. (1994). *A whole new life.* New York: Atheneum.

Lesson 7: Changing Thoughts and Feelings

Burns, D. (1980). *Feeling good.* New York: William.

Ellis, A., & Harper, R. (1975). *A new guide to rational living.* North Hollywood, CA: Wilshire Books.

Seligman, M. (1991). *Learned optimism.* New York: Knopf.

Lesson 8: Gaining Self-Confidence

McKay, M., & Fanning, P. (2000). *Self-esteem: A proven program of cogntive techniques for assessing, improving, and maintaining your self-esteem.* Oakland, CA: New Harbinger.

Taylor, S. (1999). *Living well with a hidden disability: Transcending doubt and shame and reclaiming your life.* Oakland, CA: New Harbinger.

Thorn, B. E. (2004). *Cognitive therapy for chronic pain.* New York: Guilford Press.

Lesson 9: Putting It All Together

Alberti, R. E., & Emmons, M. I. (1990). *Your perfect right: A guide to assertive living.* San Luis Obispo, CA: Impact Publications.

Brach, T. (2003). *Radical self-acceptance.* New York: Bantam.

Butler, P. (1976). *Self-assertion for women.* San Francisco: HarperCollins.

Cloud, H. (2003). *Changes that heal.* Grand Rapids, MI: Zonderman.

Lesson 10: The Importance of Maintenance and "Setbacks"

Benson, H., & Stuart, E. (1993). *The wellness book: The comprehensive guide to maintaining health and treating stress-related illness.* Secaucus, NJ: Birch Lane Press.

Cowles, J. (1993). *Pain relief! How to say "no" to acute, chronic, and cancer pain.* New York: Mastermedia.

Research Supporting This Pain Management Program

General

Compas, B. E., et al. (1998). Sampling empirically-supported psychological treatments for health psychology: Smoking, chronic pain, cancer, and bulimia nervosa. *Journal of Consulting and Clinical Psychology, 66,* 89–112.

Latham, J., & Davis, B. D. (1994). The socioeconomic impact of chronic pain. *Disability and Rehabiliation, 16,* 39–44.

Lawrence, R. C., et al. Estimates of the prevalence of selected arthritis and musculoskeletal diseases in the U.S. *Journal of Rheumatology, 16,* 427–441.

LeFort, S. M., et al. (1998). Randomized controlled trial of a community-based psychoeducation program for the self-management of chronic pain. *Pain, 74,* 297–306.

Morley, S., et al. (1999). Systematic review and meta-analysis of randomized controlled trials of cognitive behavior therapy for chronic pain in adults, excluding headache. *Pain, 80,* 1–13.

National Institutes of Health Technology Assessment Panel on Integration of Behavioral and Relaxation Approaches into the Treatment of Chronic Pain and Insomnia. (1996). Integration of behavioral and relaxation approaches into the treatment of chronic pain and insomnia. *Journal of the American Medical Association, 276,* 313–318.

Raj, P. P. (1990). Pain relief: Fact or fancy? *Regional Anesthesia, 15,* 157–169.

Scheer, S. J. (1997). Randomized controlled trials in industrial low back pain. Part 3. Subacute/chronic pain interventions. *Archives of Physical Medicine and Rehabilitation, 78,* 414–423.

Turk, D., & Gatchel, R. (Eds.). (2002). *Psychological approaches to pain management* (2nd ed.). New York: Guilford Press.

Turk, D. C., & Okifuji, A. (1998). Efficacy of multidisciplinary pain centers: Antidote for anecdotes. *Balliere's Clinical Anesthesia, 12,* 103–119.

Arthritis

Keefe, F. J., et al. (1996). Spouse-assisted coping skills training in the management of osteoarthritis knee pain. *Arthritis Care and Research, 9,* 279–291.

Leibing, E., et al. (1999). Cognitive–behavioral treatment in unselected rheumatoid arthritis outpatients. *Clinical Journal of Pain, 15,* 58–66.

Lorig, K. R., et al. (1993). Evidence suggesting that health education for self-management in patients with chronic arthritis has sustained health benefits while reducing health care costs. *Arthritis & Rheumatism, 36,* 439–446.

Parker, J. C., et al. (1995). Effects of stress management on clinical outcomes in rheumatoid arthritis. *Arthritis & Rheumatism, 38,* 1807–1818.

Sharpe, L., et al. (2001). A blind, randomized, controlled trials of cognitive-behavioral intervention for patients with recent onset rheumatoid arthritis: Preventing psychological and physical morbidity. *Pain, 89,* 275–283.

Sinclair, V. G., et al. (1998). Effects of a cognitive–behavioral intervention for women with rheumatoid arthritis. *Research in Nursing and Health, 21,* 315–326.

Back Pain

Alaranta, H., et al. (1994). Intensive physical and psychosocial training program for patients with chronic low back pain: A controlled clinical trial. *Spine, 19,* 1339–1349.

Basler, H.-D., et al. (1997). Incorporation of cognitive–behavioral treatment in the medical care of chronic low back pain patients. A controlled randomized study in German pain treatment centers. *Patient Education and Counseling, 31,* 113–124.

Boden, S. D., et al. (1990). Abnormal magnetic-resonance scans of the lumbar spine in asymptomatic subjects. *Journal of Bone and Joint Surgery, 72-A,* 403–408.

Deyo, R. A. (1986). The early diagnostic evaluation of patients with low back pain. *Journal of General Internal Medicine, 1,* 328–338.

Hasenbring, M., et al. (1999). The efficacy of a risk-factor based cognitive-behavioral intervention and electromyographic biofeedback in patients with acute sciatic pain. An attempt to prevent chronicity. *Spine, 24,* 2525–2535.

Jensen, I. B., & Bodin, L. (1998). Multimodal cognitive-behavioral treatment for workers with chronic spinal pain: A matched cohort study with an 18-month follow-up. *Pain, 67,* 35–44.

Jensen, M. C., et al. (1994). Magnetic resonance imaging of the lumbar spine in people with back pain. *New England Journal of Medicine, 331,* 69–73.

Moore, J. E., et al. (2000). A randomized trial of cognitive–behavioral program for enhancing back pain self care in primary care setting. *Pain, 88,* 145–153.

Wiesel, S. E., et al. (1984). A study of computer-assisted tomography. 1. The incidence of positive CAT scans in an asymptomatic group of patients. *Spine, 9,* 549–551.

Occupational Overuse/Cumulative Trauma/Repetitive Strain Injury

Feuerstein, M., et al. (1998). Multidisciplinary rehabilitation of chronic work-related upper extremity disorders: Long term effects. *Journal of Occupational Rehabilitation, 35,* 396–403.

Fibromyalgia

Goldenberg, D. L. (1987). Fibromyalgia syndrome. An emerging but controversial condition. *Journal of the American Medical Association, 257,* 2782–2787.

Nielson, W., et al. (1997). Outpatient cognitive–behavioral treatment of fibromyalgia: Impact on pain response and health status. *Pain Research & Management, 2,* 145–150.

Turk, D. C., et al. (1998). Interdisciplinary treatment for fibromyalgia syndrome: Clinical and statistical significance. *Arthritis Care and Research, 11,* 185–194.

Turk, D. C., et al. (1998). Differential responses by psychosocial subgroups of fibromyalgia syndrome patients to an interdisciplinary treatment. *Arthritis Care and Research, 11,* 397–404.

Headache

Basler, H.-D., et al. (1996). Cognitive-behavioral therapy for chronic headache at German pain centers. *International Journal of Rehabilitation and Health, 2,* 235–252.

Holroyd, K. A., et al. (1991). A comparison of pharmacological (amitriptyline HCl) and nonpharmacological (cognitive–behavioral) therapies for chronic tension headaches. *Journal of Consulting and Clinical Psychology, 59,* 121–133.

Mosley, T. H., et al. (1995). Treatment of tension headache in the elderly: A controlled evaluation of relaxation training and relaxation combined with cognitive–behavioral therapy. *Journal of Clinical Geropsychology, 1,* 175–188.

Osterhaus, S. O., et al. (1997). A behavioral treatment of young migrainous and nonmigrainous headache patients: Prediction of treatment success. *International Journal of Behavioral Medcine, 4,* 378–396.

Penzien, D., et al. (1990). Drug vs. behavioral treatment of migraine: Long-acting propranolol vs. home-based self-management training. *Headache, 30,* 300.

Scharff, L., et al. (1994). Interdisciplinary outpatient group treatment of intractable headache. *Headache, 34,* 73–78.

Stewart, W. F., et al. (1991). Prevalence of migraine headache in the United States: Relation to age, income, race, and other sociodeomgraphic factors. *Journal of the American Medical Association, 267,* 64–69.

Irritable Bowel Syndrome

Van Dulmen, A. M., et al. (1996). Cognitive–behavioral group therapy for irritable bowel syndrome: Effects and long-term follow-up. *Psychosomatic Medicine, 58,* 508–514.

Musculoskeletal Pain (Mixed)

Haldorsen, E. M., et al. (1998). Multimodal cognitive-behavioral treatment of patients sick-listed for musculoskeletal pain. *Scandinavian Journal of Rheumatology, 27,* 16–25.

Mixed Chronic Pain Syndromes

Becker, N. N., et al. (2000). Treatment outcome of chronic non-malignant pain patients managed in a Danish multidisciplinary pain centre compared to general practice: A randomized controlled trial. *Pain, 84,* 203–211.

Williams, A. C., et al. (1996). Inpatient vs. outpatient pain management: Results of a randomized controlled trial. *Pain, 66,* 13–22.

Noncardiac Chest Pain

Van Peski-Oosterbaan, A. S., et al. (1999). Cognitive change following cognitive behavioural therapy for non-cardiac chest pain. *Psychotherapy and Psychosomatics, 68,* 214–220.

Van Peski-Oosterbaan, A. S., et al. (1999). Cognitive-behavioral therapy for noncardiac chest pain: A randomized trial. *American Journal of Medicine 106,* 424–429.

Pelvic Pain

Peters, A. A. W., et al. (1991). A randomized clinical trial to compare two different approaches in women with chronic pelvic pain. *Obstetrics and Gynecology, 77,* 740–748.

Sickle Cell Disease

Thomas, V. J., et al. (1999). Cognitive–behaviour therapy for the management of sickle cell disease pain: An evaluation of a community-based intervention. *British Journal of Health Psychology, 4,* 209–229.

Temporomandibular Disorders

Dworkin, S. F., et al. (1994). Brief group cognitive–behavioral intervention for temporomandibular disorders. *Pain, 59,* 175–187.

Turk, D. C., et al. (1993). Effects of intraoral appliance and biofeedback/stress management along and in combination in treating pain and depression in patients with temporomandibular disorders. *Journal of Prosthetic Dentistry, 70,* 158–164.

Whiplash Injury (Neck and Shoulder Pain) Following Motor Vehicle Accidents

Vendrig, L., et al. (2002). Treatment of whiplash-associated disorders. In D. C. Turk & R. J. Gatchel (Eds.), *Psychological approaches to pain management* (2nd ed., pp. 417–437). New York: Guilford Press.

Index

About the Authors

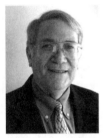

Dr. Dennis C. Turk has been involved in the assessment and treatment of people with various chronic pain conditions for over 25 years. He is the John and Emma Bonica Professor of Anesthesiology and Pain Research and director of the Fibromyalgia Research Center at the University of Washington in Seattle. Dr. Turk has published more than 380 articles and chapters in scholarly journals and books. In addition, he has written or edited 12 volumes on different aspects of pain and chronic illness including *Health, Illness and Families*; *Handbook of Pain Assessment*; and *Bonica's Management of Pain*. He is an advisor to the National Fibromyalgia Association and the American Chronic Pain Association, both groups of people with chronic pain and their families. Dr. Turk is currently the president of the American Pain Society and editor-in-chief of *The Clinical Journal of Pain*.

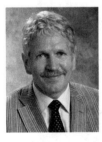

Dr. Frits Winter is head of his own pain clinic near Eindhoven in the Netherlands. Dr Winter was president of the Dutch chapter of the International Association for the Study of Pain 1994–2002. He has been involved in pain management throughout his long academic career and is the author of several self-help books, including his best-selling book *De Pijn de Baas*, (*How to Beat Pain, 7th Edition*). This book has become a standard resource in Dutch pain management programs. Dr. Winter is a teacher of postgraduate courses at the University of Groningen in Tilburg, the Netherlands, and has taught postgraduate courses at the University of Djakarta and Soerabaja in Indonesia.